A Child's Teacher

Carolyn,
Thanks so
much for
my childhood
dream true.
you did an
amazing job.
Best wishes.
:.) Nal Nelvin

A Child's Teacher

A Story of Hope

VAL MELVIN

Foreword by Mary Sue Humphrey

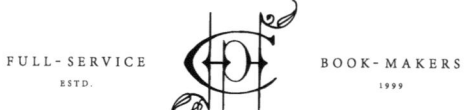

FULL-SERVICE   BOOK-MAKERS

ESTD.   1999

To Mama,

who has always been my ears when I couldn't hear,

and my voice when I couldn't speak.

Contents

Foreword

Teachers hope they make a difference in a child's life. But, sometimes, a child will make a difference in the teacher's life. Val was that child.

He was a blessing to teach. He was inquisitive and special. I enjoyed teaching him when he was in my class.

He had a unique bond with me and my family. He often stayed with us, especially on weekends when he could not go home, or when it snowed.

I am very proud of Val and his success.

Mary Sue Humphrey
Eagles Hall Teacher
Eastern North Carolina School for the Deaf

Val Melvin, Our Son

Val was born without many of the physical attributes that most of us take for granted. His physical condition at birth was so critical that we were advised: "If he makes it through the night, he will be airlifted to Duke at dawn, but his condition is very critical and you need to accept it." The doctor was as gentle as he could be, but candid in his appraisal of the situation. Val was born without inner or outer ears, and two small tags were on his cheeks that could not be explained. A lower mandible was absent; no lower jaw bone, muscle, or blood supply was present. There was no passageway for nourishment and an artificial airway had to be created. It was a temporary solution to a critical problem; the doctors needed to create a way to receive oxygen to the lungs and food to the stomach. The doctors and hospital staff stayed at his side though the night as he struggled to maintain life.

When the attending physician left my wife's side, we knelt in prayer and promised God that if our new son lived, we would walk beside him for the duration of our lives.

After multiple surgical procedures, Val, at age five, wanted to enter school, and a series of tests and evaluations revealed his capability to excel in educational studies. He had neither heard nor spoken a word in his young life, and his physical appearance was a work in progress, but behind his eyes was the desire to excel in anything that he would be involved with.

The superintendent of the Eastern North Carolina School for the Deaf, after a careful review of Val's constant medical needs and his test scores, made the decision to allow his enrollment, where he would remain on campus Monday through Friday for instruction.

The story you will read, written by Val, relates some of his challenges during his second year at ENCSD, and problems he faced as someone a little different. It is a chapter in the life of a special child who, with the help of a compassionate and wise teacher, recognized his potential to change the attitudes and feelings of other students.

The boy that they thought had severe learning disabilities because of his physical limitations, would prove them wrong and one day be inducted into the National Honor Society. He would go on to attain a college degree in computer science and programming and become employed by the North Carolina Department of Revenue, and he has, to date, never heard nor spoken one word.

The events in this story occurred as presented, and is a factual account of how a child with a positive attitude and strong faith can change the adverse behavior of other people; eliminate bullying, and develop life-long friendships with only a smile, a hug, and a handshake.

Fallon and Betty Melvin
Val's parents

Introduction

A Child's Teacher: A Story of Hope is about a caring and loving teacher, who helped her deaf student with a hole in his neck learn, and helped her students trust him. It is based on my true story, as a seven-year-old boy with my teacher, Mrs. Humphrey during my second year at ENCSD in 1976-77.

I began to write this book after watching the French film called *Marie's Story*, which is about a nun named Sister Marguerite (played by Isabelle Carré), who helps a blind and deaf girl, Marie Heurtin (played by Ariana Rivoire, who is deaf in real life), come out of her darkness and to communicate. It is based on the true story about Marie Heurtin and was filmed in France. Marie is considered the French Helen Keller. It brought back memories of Mrs. Humphrey and me as a kid. I thank the French director, Jean-Pierre Améris, for bringing *Marie's Story* into my life. It was heartwarming and it made me cry. I would have been unable to write this book if it was not for *Marie's Story*.

I wanted to write *A Child's Teacher: A Story of Hope* because I don't want anyone to bully children with birth defects. Children need to be nice to them and respect them.

Let me tell you about myself. My name is Val Melvin. My real name is Billie Fallon Melvin III, and my parents gave me the nickname Val when I was six weeks old. I was born with no ears and recessed jaws, and was sent to Duke Hospital because I had a difficult time breathing. The doctors inserted a tracheotomy (trach), to help me breath, and kept me in ICU.

My parents went to Duke Hospital and fought to take me home. The doctors made the decision to send a personal nurse to teach my parents how to take care of me. I lived in Rockingham, North Carolina for my first four years. My parents and my older brother, Alan, learned sign language because I was born deaf. I got a lot of support and love from my family and the people in Rockingham. In 1973, we moved to New Bern to be close to my paternal grandmother, who was dying. I went to Greenville for a deaf program, and they told my parents to enroll me in the Eastern North Carolina School for the Deaf in Wilson, North Carolina.

When I was six years old, I began school at ENCSD and the first building I lived in was Eagles Hall. My teacher was Ann Barnes, she taught kindergarten prep II. The principal was Sandra Simmons, and the dorm director was Thelma Cole. Miss Bass was my houseparent. The children stared at me because I had a hole in my neck, so they thought I was different from them. The staff worked hard to make them be nice to me.

Before I started at the school, my mother was not sure about me staying in the dorm, but the deaf school was far from New Bern. Ronald McAdams, the superintendent, looked at the suction machine and told my parents that the infirmary nurses would take care of it. He allowed them to explain to the nurses how to use a suction machine. I had to go to the infirmary to be suctioned and brush my teeth after each meal, three times every day.

During my first year, my teacher, Ann Barnes, taught me many things and had a hard time with the students who made fun of me. She felt very bad for me and invited me to spend a few days with her. She did an amazing job teaching me. The next school year, I met my new teacher, Mary Sue Humphrey.

I chose Mrs. Humphrey for my story because she worked hard to help me learn and helped my classmates trust me. I spent more time with her than I did with my other teachers. Mrs. Humphrey refused to give up on me and helped me learn after learning about my difficult birth. My parents trusted Mrs. Humphrey to teach me and became good friends with her and her husband. I had many wonderful moments with her. My favorite moment is when Humphrey made me eat pimento cheese sandwiches. She was very scared of me eating them quickly because she thought I would choke.

Some special moments with Mrs. Humphrey include meeting her husband and her sons, going to the infirmary after lunch together, telling Humphrey I loved her for the first time, spending a few days with her and her family in the summer of 1976, and when I stayed with them on a winter weekend because I was unable to be with my family during my grandfather's death. Mrs. Humphrey wanted me to stay with her and her family so she could comfort me. When I got older, I saw her sometimes and visited her and her family. She was there for my graduation, and she and her husband were there for my brother's wedding. I enjoyed having her at my 40th birthday party, and her son Thomas and his family were there as well. When I decided to write the book about us, I asked for her permission; she said she would be honored to be in the story. She was very pleased to read it and she recalled some special moments. Her husband and her sons are in the story too because they were sweet and kind to me. I felt like I had a second family when I stayed with them.

There are nine important children in the story because they were in my class with Mrs. Humphrey. There are three boys and six girls (two are black; another is Mexican). Besides Mrs. Humphrey, my classmates, and me, there are Mrs. Cole, Miss Bass, Miss Simmons, Clara Eatmon, Beth Dawson, two infirmary nurses (Barnes and Farmer), my parents, my brother Alan, Humphrey's husband and their sons (Thomas and Blaine), James Massey the school director, and Gary Farmer, my PE teacher. Beverly and Sue Dail are mentioned; Beverly (Miss Rockingham pageant queen) made her first visit to ENCSD when I was in Mrs. Eatmon's class.

I want to thank my good friend Terry Dunaway who suggested that I write a book about my life. I also took advice from my cousin's wife, Sue Jones who is a writer; I want to thank her too. I thank Melinda Wright Lanier for suggesting this beautiful title for my book. I thank my father for editing the grammar and spelling before the book was re-edited. I thank my caring and loving parents who kept fighting for me after my birth. I love my parents with all my heart because they worked hard to support me and helped me look my best after the operations. I thank Alan for being there for me when I needed him. I wish my grandmother could read this story, but I am sure she is very proud of me. I want all of you to enjoy this story, which is based on my life.

Also, I want to thank my wonderful teacher, Mary Sue Humphrey, for helping me learn. I don't know what I would have done if it wasn't for her. I love her with all my heart, and I will never forget her. Thanks to her, pimento cheese is my favorite sandwich.

Family Photo Album

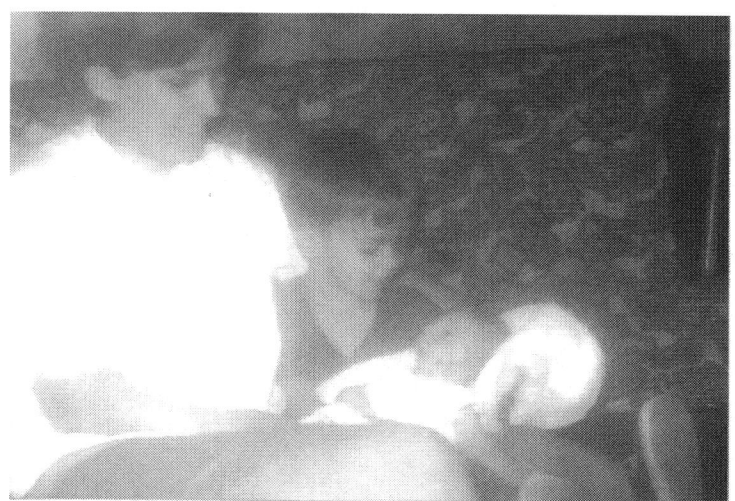

I arrived home from Duke Hospital at two months; this is the first picture of me. My brother, Alan, held me as a newborn as my mother looked on.

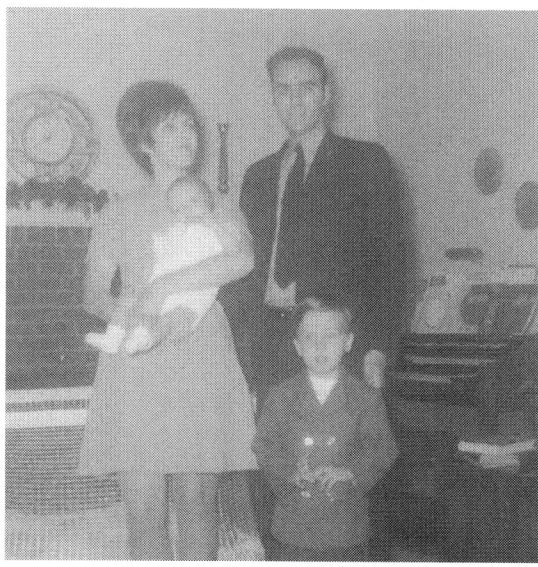

This is the first picture of the Melvin family, taken when I was three months old. This picture was taken in my paternal grandmother's house near Belgrade, North Carolina.

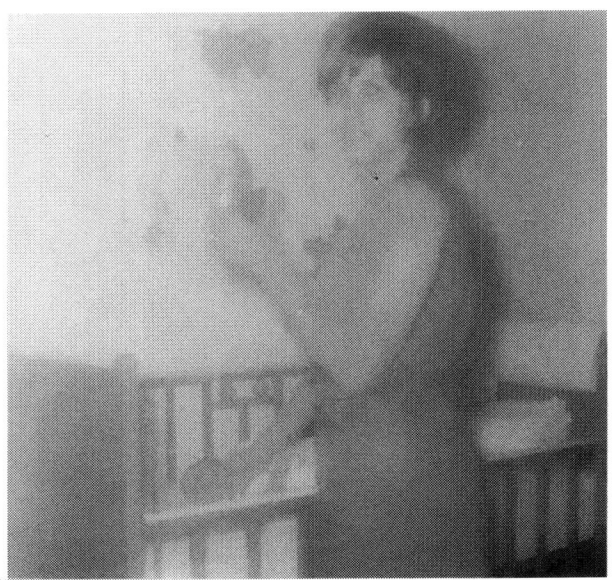

Mama learned how to feed me with a milk bottle in my room at our Rockingham home. She suffered from depression after my birth; she was determined to take care of me herself, so the doctors got a personal nurse to teach her how.

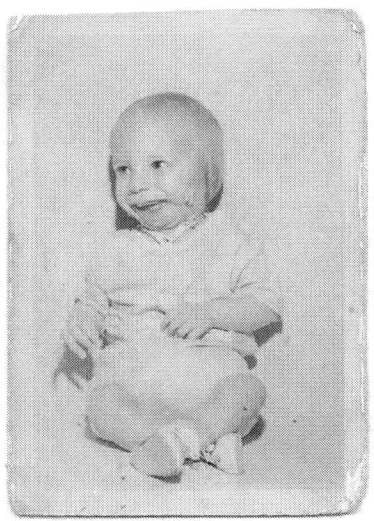

Me at six months old; I was born with recessed jaws and no ears. I had a breathing problem, so the doctor inserted a trach.

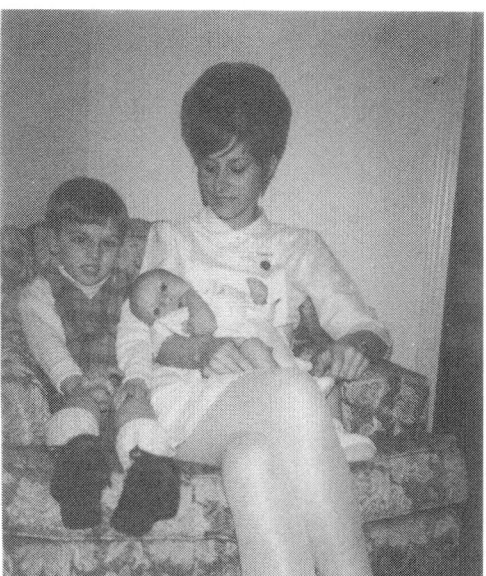

Alan, Kathy Leandro, and me, at six months old; Kathy was one of the nurses who took care of me every day. My parents asked Kathy to be my godmother at my christening in January of 1970.

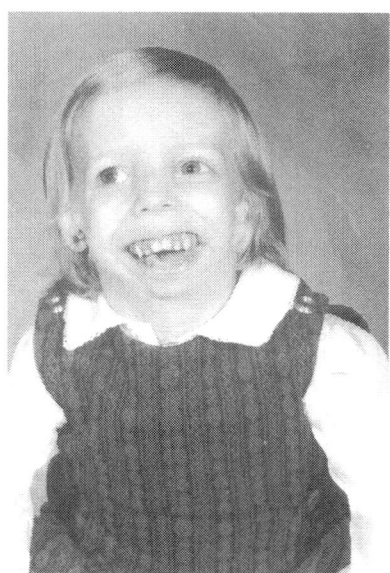

Me at three years old; Mama always hid my trach in my clothes.

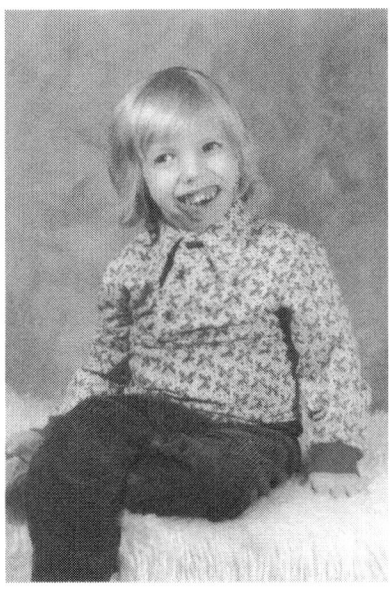

Me at four years old, when we moved to New
Bern, North Carolina, in the summer of 1973.

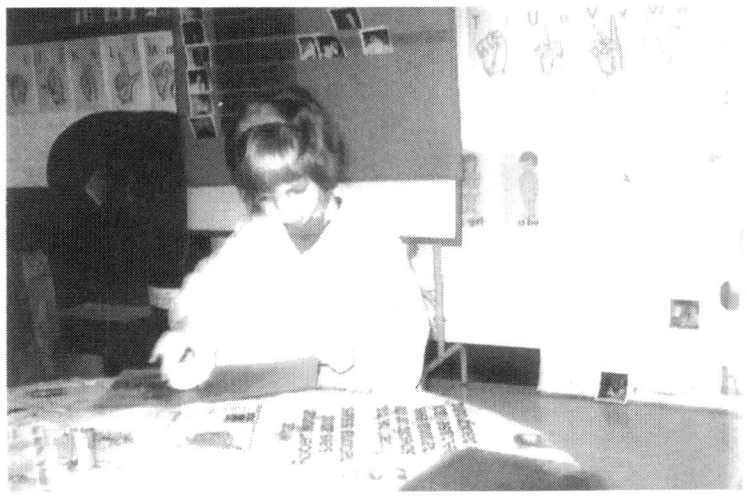

When I was five years old, my education began at the Pre-K program
for the deaf in Greenville, North Carolina, during the 1974-1975 year.

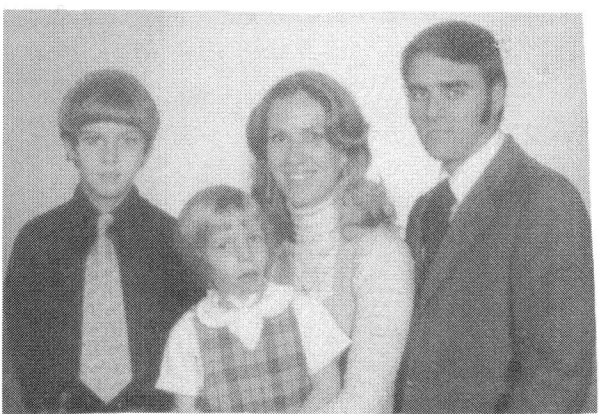

This family picture was taken when I was four years old. My family and I moved from Rockingham to New Bern, my childhood hometown, in June 1973. My father began to preach at the Methodist Church in Pamlico County.

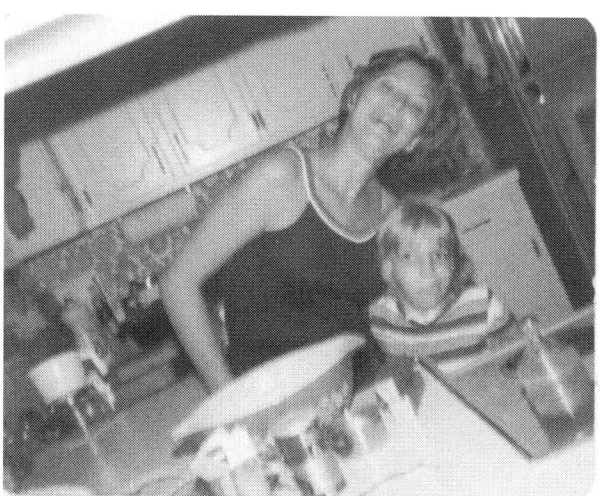

Beverly Long and me, at age 7, at my Red Fox Road home in New Bern, during the summer of 1977. She was my first babysitter, but she later moved to Wilson. As you can see in this picture, I was not happy because my jaws were wired shut after another operation. Beverly gave me a big hug and showed me her braces to make me feel better.

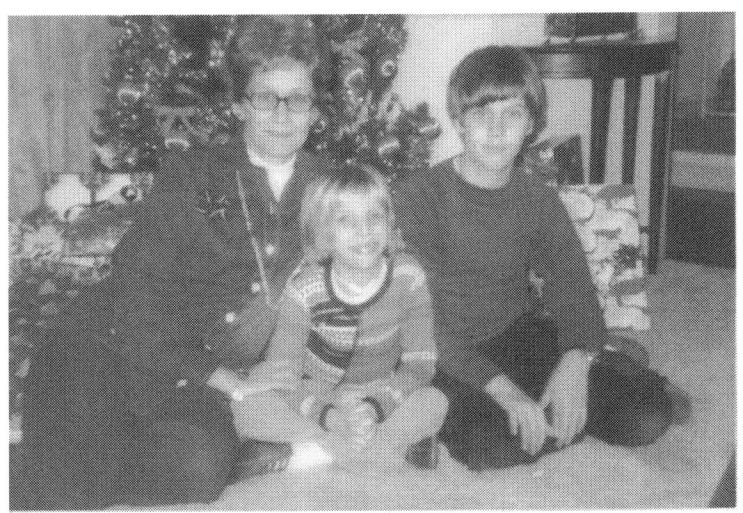

Grandma Merle Woodburn, Alan, and me (age 8), at Christmas 1977.

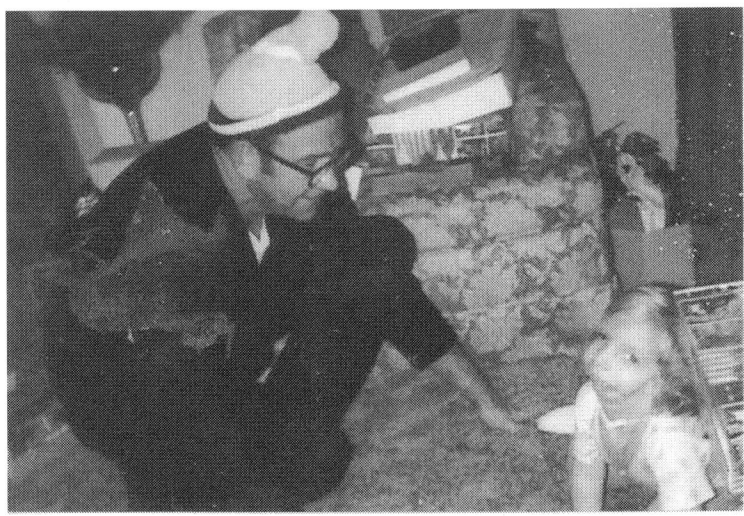

Grandpa Maurice Woodburn and me (age 4), on Christmas 1973, at our Steeple Chase Road home in New Bern. He made me laugh hard when he wore my hat. This is my favorite picture of Grandpa and me.

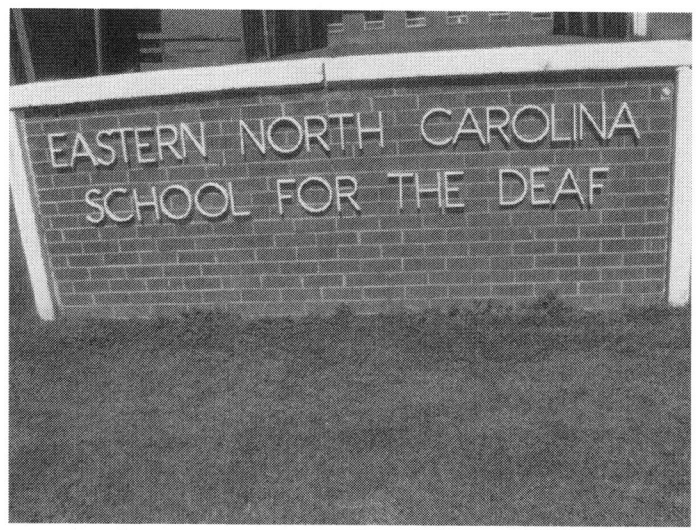

Eastern North Carolina School for the Deaf in Wilson, North Carolina, was established in 1964; the first superintendent was Ronald McAdams. I enrolled in ENCSD in August 1975, and stayed there until I graduated on May 27, 1988.

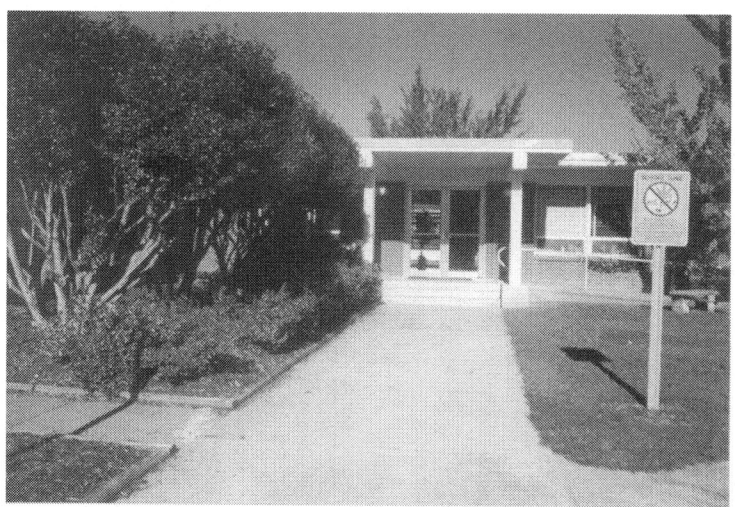

Eagles Hall was the first dorm I lived in; I stayed there for three years before moving to Vestal Hall. I have many fond memories there.

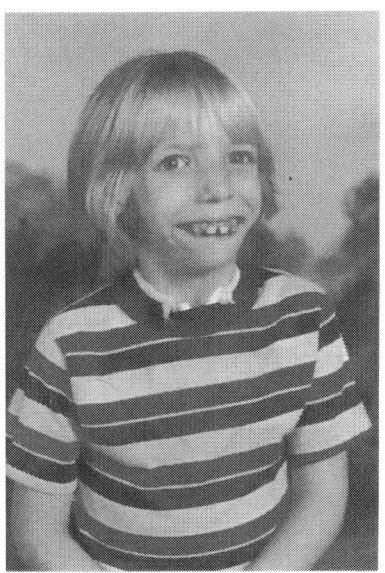

The first ENCSD picture of me when I was six years old. I was in Ann Barnes' class for kindergarten prep II. I tried to hide my trach in my shirt because I didn't like anyone staring at me.

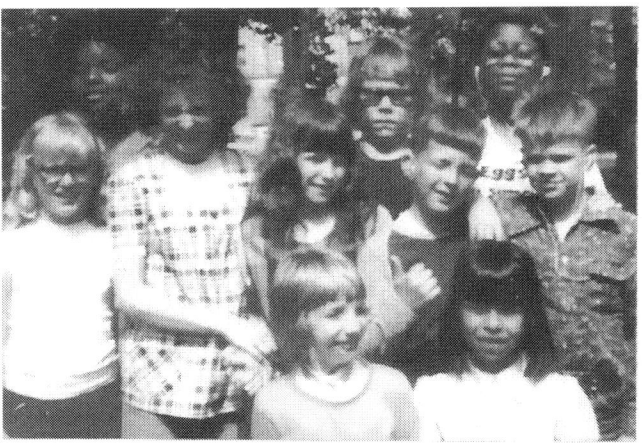

My nine classmates and me in Raleigh, North Carolina, for a field trip. Front row: me and Carolina Enriquez. Middle row: Traci Baines, Kathy Yott, Cindy Williams, Stephen Phillips, and Matthew Halstead. Back row: Corie Jackson, Junior Harrison and Cassandra Porter.

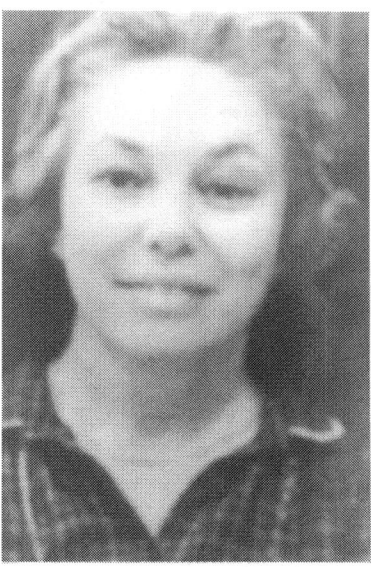

Mary Sue Humphrey was my teacher for kindergarten prep III. It was my second year at ENCSD (1976-77). She had a hard time with me at first, but we eventually grew closer and she helped me learn. She was married to CW Humphrey and has two sons, Thomas and Blaine.

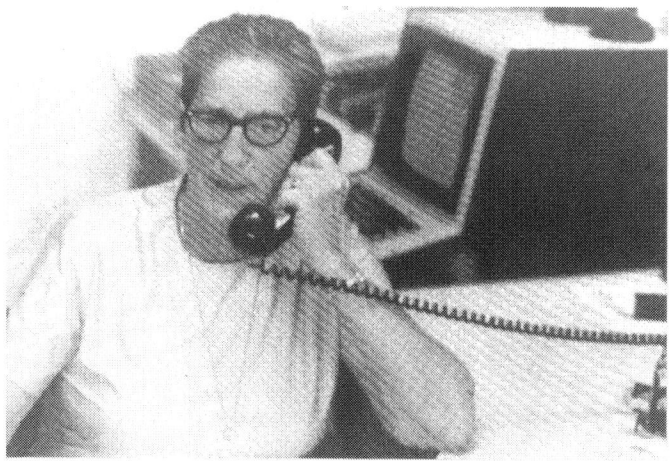

Thelma Cole was the dorm director at Eagles Hall, and she was the first staff member I trusted when I began school. I had a hard time with my parents leaving me alone, so Cole comforted me by giving me cookies and milk. She treated me like the son she never had; I visited her office after my graduation.

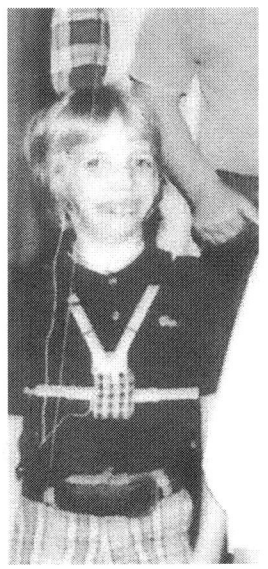

Me at age 8; I was uncomfortable wearing my hearing aid.

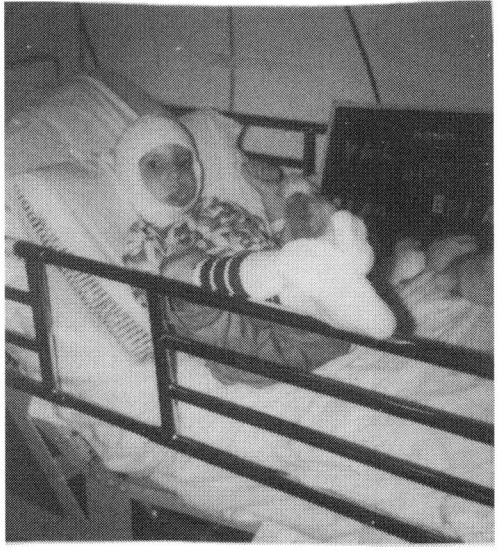

Me at age seven in Duke Hospital for my ears and jaws operations. I had many operations at Duke Hospital, until 1986 when I went to Boston. I then went to the Carolina Medical Center in Charlotte, North Carolina. Thanks to that doctor, my face looks very good and I got a new left ear.

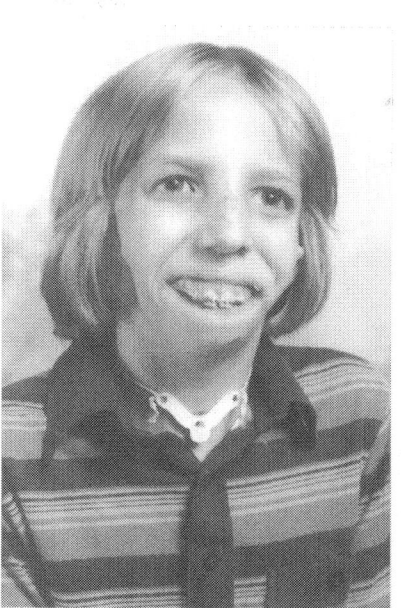

I was in the fourth grade, this is one of the last pictures of me wearing the trach.

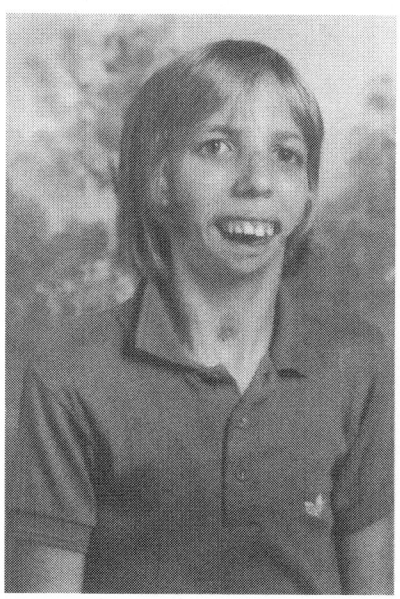

I was in the seventh grade; I still had a hole in my neck.

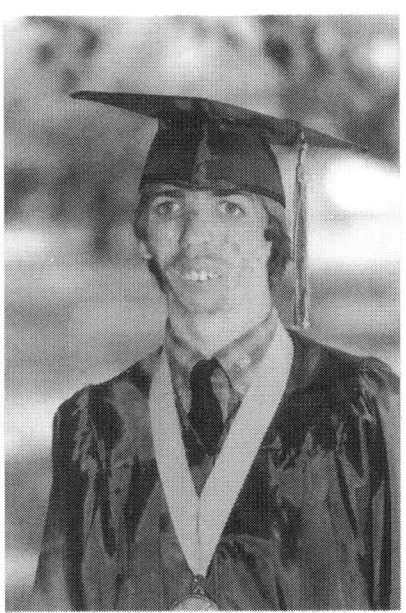

Me at eighteen years old, I graduated from ENCSD with a high school diploma on May 27, 1988. I was a member of the National Honor Society.

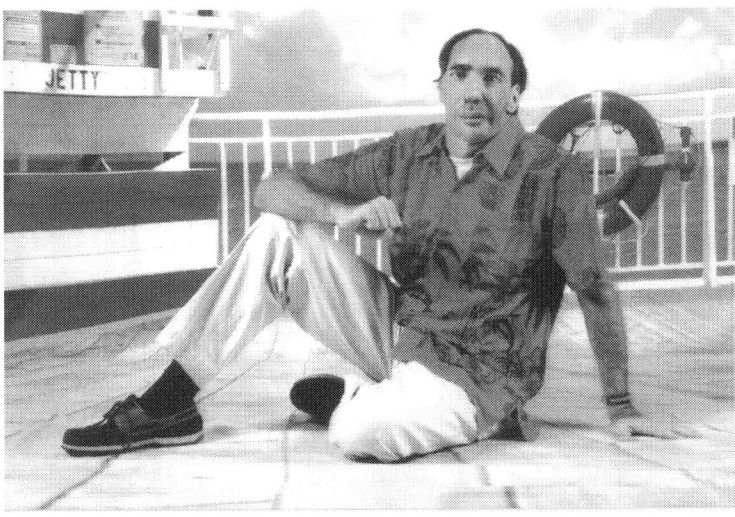

This is a current picture of me. I am very blessed to look better after many operations throughout the years. I thank my parents for their love and support.

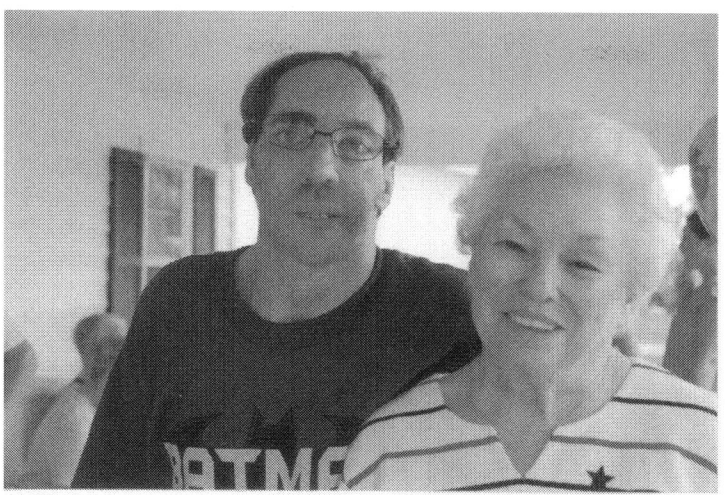

Mrs. Humphrey and me at White Lake for my 40th birthday. We discussed many fond memories. Her older son, Thomas, and his family were also there.

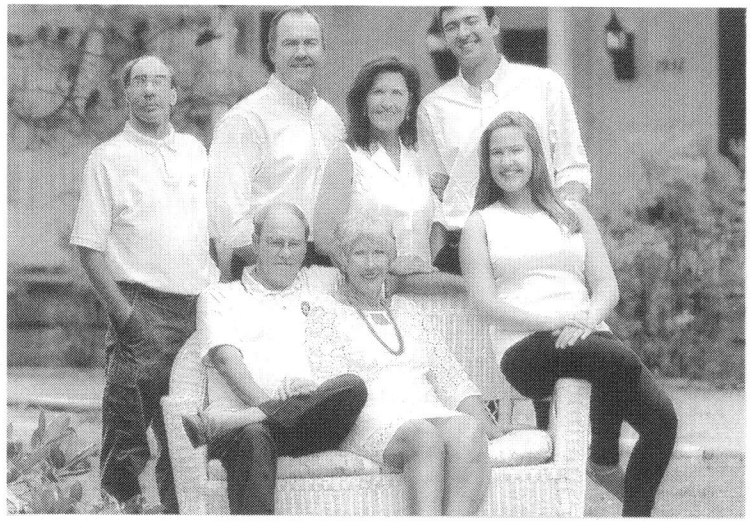

The Melvin family at White Lake in 2014 for my parents' 50th anniversary. Back row: me, my brother, Alan; sister-in-law, Allison; and nephew, Joseph. Front row: my father, Fallon; mother, Betty; and niece, Emily.

Acknowledgments

In loving memory of
Traci Baines
Thelma Cole
Grandpa Maurice and Grandma Merle
CW Humphrey
Clara Eatmon
James Massey
I wish all of you could read this story and I love all of you!

In the caring and loving honor of
Mama, Papa, Alan, Allison, Joseph and Emily.
The best teacher, Mary Sue Humphrey.
Terry Dunaway, who suggested I write this book,
Melinda Wright Lanier, who gave me
the beautiful title for this book, and
Sue Jones, who gave me advice about writing the book.

I would like to thank Sandra Fox,
my interpreter and dear friend,
who helped me with the grammar and the spelling.

Thanks so much for your support! I love you all so much.

Prologue

On July 30, 1969 at 10:37pm, I was born to Billie Fallon Melvin, Jr, and his wife, Betty Woodburn Melvin, at Richmond County Memorial Hospital in Rockingham, North Carolina. My parents were looking forward to seeing me and holding me, but the next day, I was transferred to Duke Hospital for observation and diagnosis. My parents were told that I had a hole in my neck, recessed jaws, and no ears. I was also deaf. They were very upset to find out about my birth defects, and my mother kept asking my father to drive her to Duke Hospital to see me. My parents named me after my father and my paternal grandfather who died a few months before I was born. Although my real name is Billie Fallon Melvin III, my parents were considering a nickname as I was rushed to Duke Hospital.

My mother was upset because she wanted to see and hold me before I was transferred. The doctor advised against my mother's wish. My mother told the doctor that I was beautiful and was God's gift to her. The doctor said he had no choice and suggested my parents go to Duke Hospital to talk to the doctors about me. My older brother, Alan, then two years old, was with my maternal grandparents at our Rockingham home. My mother didn't know what to do. She was anxious to get out of the hospital and go to Duke to see me.

On August 5, my parents went to Duke to spend two weeks learning to take care of me. My mother visited the intensive care nursery every four hours to learn to feed me. The first time my mother visited the nursery, she got upset as she saw the many deformed children and learned how she would have to feed me. She returned to the motel, saying she would never be able to do it. My parents stayed up that night thinking and praying; the decision was to take me home. The next morning, my parents resolved to be strong for me and were determined to learn.

The attending physicians at Duke Hospital were supportive: Dr. William DeMaria was the Head Pediatrician. He was a very compassionate man, a very good friend to the family, and always there for emotional support.

My plastic surgeon, was a very good doctor, but his bedside manner left a lot to be desired. He didn't feel the need to keep the family fully informed, and was very distant. No compassion was shown and he was very negative.

Dr. Farmer, ENT was also a very good doctor and he felt like family. He felt emotional adjustment was very important. He was easy to talk to and he didn't rush conversations concerning the patient.

At the end of August 1969, I returned home after the doctors at Duke were comfortable with the feeding technique. Family doctors advised in the care of the emotional needs of our family. The health nurse came by once a week to monitor my care; my mother did very well with feeding, but worried because I always seemed to be hungry. I was restless and wanted to nurse my mother, but she was determined to teach me to drink from a bottle. This was a very hard and trying time, but I did learn. My mother gave me cereal with the milk though a bottle, but continued tube feeding to insure I was getting enough nourishment. Alan was very happy to meet his little brother, but he was too young to understand why I stayed in the hospital for so long. He still loved me.

As time passed, the pressure grew and sleep was rare. My mother was nervous and depressed, but covered it with a strong image. Luckily, family doctors saw me though it all and recommended a private duty nurse for the 11-7 shift every night. Money was limited, but insurance paid for it. They got an LPN, Mrs. Patton, who was very good with me. She rocked me a lot and loved hot tea.

My mother took me out to the local hospital once a month, and Dr. Durclin took me to the OR to insert a clean trach. Later, when mother felt confident, she could do it at home, but was very nervous the first time. She lived with the constant fear of losing me.

My father, Billie Fallon Melvin, Jr., is the son of Billie Fallon Melvin and Glennie Stroud and was born in McRae, GA. He is called Fallon. He and his parents moved to Wilmington where his younger brother, Lewis, was born. His parents divorced when he was young. My great grandfather, Ralph Preston Melvin, ran a resort in White Lake until he died. Then my grandfather and his siblings continued the work. The brothers sold the land to the Clearwater Camp in 1964.

My father and my uncle grew up near Maysville, North Carolina with their mother, but they stayed with their father every summer.

My mother, Betty Rice Woodburn, is the daughter of U.S. Army Sergeant, Thomas Maurice Woodburn, and his wife, Merle Jane Rice. My mother was born in Fayetteville and had two younger sisters, Tommy and Lennie. Their family used to live in Germany, when my grandpa was in World War II, but they moved back to the United States, and lived in many different places.

My parents met each other for the first time at White Lake. My mother used to work at the Goldston Beach sandwich shop, and met my father at the White Lake dance. My father went to East Carolina, while my mother went to the school of cosmetology. They got engaged before President Kennedy was killed and they got married in Tabernacle Methodist church on July 19, 1964 two days before my father's 23rd birthday. They went to Wrightsville Beach for their honeymoon. Their first home was a mobile home in Fayetteville where my father taught history at Massey High School. My parents later moved their mobile home to Wilmington, where my father worked at JC Penny and my mother worked at the courthouse. He later decided to work for Carolina Power and Light.

Their first son was born in Wilmington, North Carolina. They named him Jonathan Alan Melvin and called him by his middle name. My parents and Alan lived in the trailer at Whiteville, North Carolina. They later moved to Kinston, but they lived there only a year before moving to Rockingham, North Carolina. The first house they lived in was 716 Sycamore Lane. One year later, I was born.

After I came home from Duke Hospital, I had many doctors' appointments. The personal nurse had to stay in our house for tube feeding until my parents learned to take care of me. The nurse left, but visited our house often to check on how I was doing. My parents had a hard time explaining to Alan why I got more attention than he did. He was too young to understand, but he never complained. My doctors and nurses called me Billie, but when I was six weeks old, my parents made the decision to call me Val. It came from my father's nickname by his college buddies. I didn't know about my real name until I noticed it written down in Duke Hospital. Because I was deaf, my parents were forced to learn sign language to communicate with me. Alan learned sign language when he started school in 1971.

People in Rockingham supported my parents in keeping me and wanted to meet me. Another nurse helped my mother take care of me; her name was Kathy. She became my godmother, and I called her Aunt Kathy.

In 1971, I had my first operation at Duke Hospital. I was very scared of the operation, especially the IV. I spent a few months there because I was unable to chew due to my recessed jaws. The doctor gave my parents some information about foods I could eat. I ate soft foods like applesauce, mashed potatoes, and Rice Krispies. I later went to Duke Hospital for my hearing test and got a new hearing aid, but I didn't like it.

I started to crawl when I was a toddler and I stood for the first time when I was three years old. My parents kept waiting for me to walk, but I was not ready for a while. During this time, Alan and I had a babysitter named Beverly Long. She went to Duke Hospital to learn how to take care of me. She was like a second mother to me. We had a very special bond.

We traveled a lot to see my grandparents in Fayetteville, North Carolina and went to White Lake to see relatives. I was unable to swim at White Lake, but my parents hauled me around. By age three, I had learned sign language like mama, papa, drink, eat, and sleep. Beverly surprised me by communicating with me using sign language. My parents talked about sending me to the deaf school when I got older.

After living in Rockingham, North Carolina, for my first four years, my father decided to move us to New Bern, North Carolina to be close to his mother who was dying. Some people in Rockingham were very sad to see us leave. They had a farewell party for us. Some of the men helped my father move the stuff to New Bern and some of the women at Rockingham kept kissing me with their lipstick, especially Beverly. Alan said goodbye to his friends at school. I was too young to understand about moving day, but I asked my mother if we would see Aunt Kathy and Beverly again. It took a few days to move to New Bern. Our house was at 2205 Steeplechase Drive. It had three bedrooms and two bathrooms. I still slept in a crib, until I was ready for a bed. My father had his office in the living room and he began to preach at Pamlico County Methodist Church. I was very shy with people, but soon became comfortable around new friends. I met a deaf man at Stonewall North Carolina, his name was Asa Gatlin, Jr. I sat with him when we had lunch at the church.

We visited my paternal grandmother every weekend until she passed away. I didn't understand about death. When I was five, I went to Greenville for the deaf program and met deaf children there. They were very kind and sweet to me. We played together and made pudding, I had a great time. My parents were told that I would need to enroll in the Eastern North Carolina School for the Deaf in Wilson, North Carolina, so my father made an appointment to meet the superintendent, Mr. Ronald McAdams, for my enrollment.

I was six years old and was very nervous to meet Mr. McAdams. The man looked at me and asked my parents, point blank, what happened to the hole in my neck. He didn't mean to ask them so bluntly. My father explained my birth and my special needs.

Ronald McAdams realized that I was very special and told my parents that he would be happy to enroll me at ENCSD. Also, he told them I would stay in the dorm because New Bern was an hour and half from Wilson. My mother was not sure about me staying in the dorm because I needed to be suctioned three times each day. My father pulled the suction machine from the car and showed it to him. Ronald suggested that the infirmary nurses could take care of cleaning my trach. Also, my parents told Ronald that I wouldn't ride the bus home on weekends because they had to pick the suction machine up every Friday and bring it back every Sunday. Afterwards, he gave us a tour of Eagles Hall, and we met teachers and students.

I started school on August 24th. My father looked very pleased, but my mother was not comfortable about the deaf children staring at me and treating me badly. My father told her that the houseparent and the teacher would take care of me. I kept looking at my mother packing my clothes in my suitcase. Alan asked my parents if they were getting to rid of me, but they explained why I needed to go to the deaf school. They told him I would come home every weekend. He cried and hugged me. I didn't understand why I had to go there, but I knew education was important.

When I arrived at school, deaf children kept staring at me. I was uncomfortable with that. I met the dorm director named Thelma Cole, I was not sure if I trusted her, but I got along quickly with her after she gave me cake and milk. She was like a mother to me when I stayed at Eagles Hall. My parents and I met the principal; her name was Sandra Simmons. I called her Miss Simmons. She accompanied me and my parents to meet my teacher, named Ann Barnes, who was very sweet and kind to me.

I ran away from the classroom when my parents left, but Mrs. Cole grabbed me and comforted me. Mrs. Cole took me to the infirmary in Woodard Hall where the suction machine was. Jean Barnes read the instruction manual and suctioned me and cleaned my teeth. Before I went to bed, I asked my houseparent for warm milk, but she didn't understand what I was saying until Mrs. Cole explained it to her. Mrs. Cole knew what to do with me because she had listened when my parents explained.

Ann Barnes taught me and my classmates in the kindergarten Prep II class. There were seven students, including me. The classroom had a restroom inside so the kids didn't have to go down the hall. She found out I loved numbers and taught me how to count, I remember counting little bears. Ann had a hard time getting her students to trust me because they thought I was different from them. They were jealous when Ann paid more attention to me than to them. They realized I was very good at numbers and finally accepted who I was.

Ann Barnes got me an "I love you" t-shirt and I thanked her. Before I left for the summer, she asked if I wanted to spend a few days with her. I told her I would love to, but I reminded her to ask my mother for permission. Ann looked very nervous about asking my mother, but I told her my mother didn't bite. Ann laughed and finally asked my mother if I could spend in few days with her and her family. My parents approved. When I stayed with Ann and her husband, their two children were out for summer camp. I was disappointed, but I realized that her daughter had a Snoopy plush and Peanuts stuff. I told her I wanted a Snoopy plush like that. She smiled and told me that my parents might get it for me one day. Ann knew I wanted to meet her two children and to go somewhere like the swimming pool and ride a horse.

Ann was a very good teacher, and she was the reason I became a Snoopy fan. That year we moved to another house at 3050 Red Fox Road. My father got his own room for an office upstairs and he moved to Riverdale Methodist Church to preach.

The next school year, I met a new teacher, Mary Sue Humphrey.

The Characters

Val Melvin	A seven-year-old deaf boy with a trach, recessed jaws, and no interior or exterior ears
May Sue Humphrey	Caring and loving Eagles Hall teacher who helps Val learn and become friends with the other students
Thelma Cole	Eagles Hall dorm director
Sandra Simmons	Eagles Hall principal
Miss Bass	Val's Eagles Hall houseparent
Beth Dawson	Eagles Hall teacher and Humphrey's best friend
Betty Melvin	Val's mother and homemaker
Fallon Melvin	Val's father and a Methodist pastor
Alan Melvin	Val's older brother; he is ten years old
CW Humphrey	Humphrey's husband
Thomas Humphrey	Humphrey's older son
Blaine Humphry	Humphrey's younger son
Maurice and Merle Woodburn	Val's maternal grandparents
Miss Ezzard	A substitute teacher

Clara Eatmon	Val's teacher after Humphrey
Carol Farmer and Jean Barnes	Infirmary nurses who clean Val's trach
Gary Farmer	PE Teacher
James Massey	Director of the Eastern North Carolina School for the Deaf

Val's Classmates

Traci Baines	A blonde haired girl who is sweet to Val after meeting his mother. Her smile is beautiful.
Junior Harrison	A boy who feels very bad for Val and becomes a good friend to him. He is the oldest in the class.
Stephen Phillips	A boy with short hair. He gives Val a hard time and later becomes his friend.
Cindy Williams	A girl with brown hair; she is always smiling.
Carolina Enrique	A small Mexican girl who is about the same size as Val.
Cassandra Porter	A black girl and the tallest in the class.
Kathy Yott	A girl with natural curls; she is almost as tall as Cassandra.
Corie Jackson	A black girl with some curls
Matthew Halstead	A nice looking boy, but very quiet

Note: *They were in Humphrey and Eatmon's classes with me. When we moved to Vestal Hall, we were separated due to our ages. Matthew, Carolina, and Corie left the deaf school while we were in Vestal Hall. Junior graduated from ENCSD in 1985. Stephen and Kathy graduated in 1986, Cassandra graduated in 1987. Cindy and Traci graduated with me in 1988*

Fade In:

Scene One: Going to the Deaf School

Val and his parents are in the car going to the school for the deaf. Val looks through the window, then turns to his mother.

VAL   *[Sign]* Mama, where are we going?

BETTY   *[Sign]* We are going to take you to the school for the deaf.

VAL   *[Sign]* School?

BETTY   *[Sign]* Yes, you will learn at the school, and you can communicate with the deaf students.

VAL   *[Sign]* Why did you bring my suitcase?

BETTY   *[Sign]* I will explain everything when we get there.

They arrive at the school in Wilson and go to Eagles Hall. Val reads the sign, "Eastern North Carolina School for the Deaf," and he looks around.

FALLON   *[Sign]* Val, here is your school. I hope you will like it.

VAL   *[Sign]* Wow!

BETTY   *[Sign]* I hope you will enjoy it.

Eagles Hall Foyer

COLE   *[Sign]* Welcome to Eagles Hall! My name is Thelma Cole. I am the dorm director. Call me Mrs. Cole.

VAL   *[Sign]* Wow, can you sign?

COLE   *[Sign]* Yes. What is your name?

VAL   *[Sign]* My name is Val.

COLE   *[Sign]* Nice name. Welcome to Eagles Hall.
                You will stay in the dorm.

VAL   *[Sign]* Dorm?

BETTY   *[Voice]* Mrs. Cole, Val doesn't know about the
                dorm. We are Val's parents.

FALLON   *(Shakes Cole's hand)* *[Voice]* Mrs. Cole, nice to
                meet you.

COLE   *[Voice]* I am glad to meet you. If you are
                looking for registration, go to the TV room.

FALLON   *[Voice]* Where do I put Val's suitcase?

COLE   *[Voice]* Follow me. We will go to the dorm
                where Val will stay.

FALLON   *[Voice]* Thanks so much!

The Melvins and Mrs. Cole go to the dorm.

Eagles Hall Dorm

MISS BASS   *[Voice]* Hello Mrs. Cole, may I help you?

COLE   *[Voice]* Hello Miss Bass, this boy will be
                staying here. His name is Val Melvin. These
                are his parents.

MISS BASS   *[Sign]* Hello Val, welcome to the dorm. I am
                your houseparent Miss Bass.

BETTY   *[Voice]* I will explain everything about him
                after meeting his teacher. Thanks!

MISS BASS	*[Voice and sign]* You're welcome, it is no problem. Val, I will see you later.
VAL	*[Sign]* Mama?
BETTY	*[Sign]* Yes, dear?
VAL	*[Sign]* Do I need to stay here?
BETTY	*[Sign]* Yes, this is your school.
VAL	*[Sign]* Why don't we go home now?
BETTY	*[Sign]* It is too far, but we will pick you up on Friday.
VAL	*[Sign]* I don't want to stay here! I want to go home!
BETTY	*(Sighs)* *[Voice]* I don't know what to do.
FALLON	*[Voice]* Don't worry, Mrs. Cole will take care of him.
SIMMONS	*[Voice]* Hello, my name is Sandra Simmons, the principal. Is your boy deaf?
BETTY	*[Voice]* Yes, his name is Val Melvin. He is nervous about going here.
SIMMONS	*[Voice]* I understand. Go register, then we will meet Val's teacher.
VAL	*(Looks at Miss Simmons)* *[Sign]* Who is this?
SIMMONS	*[Sign]* Hello, you must be Val; I am your principal, Miss Simmons. Hope you will love the school here.
VAL	*(Turns to his mama)* *[Sign]* Can we go home?

BETTY   *[Sign]* Please be quiet. We are going to meet your teacher soon.

VAL   *[Sign]* Please don't leave me alone. I want to stay with you and Papa.

BETTY   *[Voice]* Sigh!

FALLON   *[Voice]* Miss Simmons, we are done with registration. We would like to meet Val's new teacher. Her name is Mary Sue Humphrey.

SIMMONS   *[Voice]* Sure, come with me to her classroom.

FALLON   *[Voice]* Thanks so much.

VAL   *[Sign]* Mama, where are we going?

BETTY   *[Sign]* To meet your teacher. Her name is Mary Sue Humphrey. Please be nice to her.

VAL   *[Sign]* Okay. Do you want me to stay here?

BETTY   *[Sign]* I will explain everything later. Okay?

Miss Simmons escorts Val and his parents to the classroom to meet his new teacher.

Humphrey's Classroom

SIMMONS   *[Voice and sign]* Here is the Humphrey classroom. Val, I hope you like your new teacher.

Val is silent.

HUMPHREY   *[Sign]* Good afternoon, I am your teacher. My name is Mrs. Mary Sue Humphrey. You must be Val Melvin, welcome to my classroom. I am glad that I will be teaching you this year.

VAL	*[Sign]* Hello, Mrs. Humphrey.
FALLON	*[Voice]* Hello, Mrs. Humphrey! We are Val's parents. My name is Fallon Melvin, and this is my wife Betty.
HUMPHREY	*[Voice]* Hello, Mr. and Mrs. Melvin. Nice to meet you two.
BETTY	*[Sign]* Val, what do you say to Mrs. Humphrey?

Val looks at Mrs. Humphrey and hides behind his mother.

BETTY	*[Voice]* It's okay; he is shy. I am sure you two will get along well.
HUMPHREY	*[Sign]* Val, please don't be shy. I want to show you your desk.

Val looks around at his desk.

VAL	*[Sign]* I see my name on the desk.
HUMPHREY	*[Sign]* Yes, it is your desk. I am sure you will enjoy the class. Do you have your hearing aid with you?
VAL	*[Sign]* Mama has mine.
BETTY	*[Voice]* Here is his hearing aid. He will wear it tomorrow, but it is uncomfortable for him.
HUMPHREY	*[Voice to parents and sign to Val]* Don't worry, I will take care of everything. Val, you can look around here.
VAL	*[Sign]* Humphrey?
HUMPHREY	*[Sign]* Yes, Val?

VAL	*[Sign]* How many kids will be here?
HUMPHREY	*[Sign]* Ten, including you. You will meet your classmates tomorrow.
VAL	*[Sign]* Wow. Can they sign?
HUMPHREY	*[Sign]* Of course, they are deaf like you are. You can communicate with them.
VAL	*[Sign]* That's good. I like to make friends.
HUMPHREY	*[Sign]* Great, I am sure you will like the class here.
VAL	*[Sign]* May I ask you something?
HUMPHREY	*[Sign]* What is it?
VAL	*[Sign]* How far is it from home?
HUMPHREY	*[Voice]* Mr. Melvin, I think you need to explain to your son about how far home is.
FALLON	*[Sign]* Val, your home is one hour and 30 minutes from here. That's why you have to stay in the dorm.
VAL	*[Sign]* I didn't think I would stay here.
BETTY	*[Sign]* Val, you need to stay here. She will teach you new things.
VAL	*[Sign]* I want to go to school with Alan. It sounds like fun.
BETTY	*[Sign]* Listen to me, Alan goes to the hearing school. They don't use sign language to talk with you. Deaf children are here so you can make friends.

FALLON   *[Sign]* Right. We better unpack your clothes before we leave. Tell Mrs. Humphrey you will see her tomorrow.

VAL   *[Sign]* Okay. Humphrey, see you tomorrow.

HUMPHREY   *[Sign to Val and voice to his parents]* Thanks so much for coming. See you tomorrow. I am looking forward to having you. *(Turns to Mr. and Mrs. Melvin)* Nice to meet you. I will take care of your son.

BETTY   *[Voice]* Thanks so much, Mrs. Humphrey. I will see you on Friday. Have a good evening.

Eagles Hall Main Hallway

BETTY   *[Sign]* What do you think about Mrs. Humphrey?

VAL   *[Sign]* She is okay.

BETTY   *[Sign]* Val, I want you to be nice to her. You will like her someday. We better go to the dorm and unpack your clothes.

VAL   *[Sign]* Okay. Are you going to leave me here?

BETTY   *[Sign]* Oh, Val. I will pick you up on Friday. You will be with us every weekend.

VAL   *[Sign]* Who will take care of me?

BETTY   *[Sign]* Take it easy. Mrs. Cole, Miss Bass, Mrs. Humphrey, and the nurse will.

The Eagles Hall Boy's Dorm

Val and his parents go to the dorm and Betty unpacks Val's things. Val looks around the dorm as Miss Bass comes in.

MISS BASS   *[Voice]* Hello Mrs. Melvin, may I help you?

BETTY	*[Voice]* No, I am done with the clothes anyway. I need you to show me to the bathroom.
MISS BASS	*[Voice]* Sure, come on.

They go into the bathroom so Betty can see the shower and tub.

BETTY	*[Voice]* Do the kids use the showers?
MISS BASS	*[Voice]* Yes, what about Val?
BETTY	*[Voice]* I would rather Val use the tub, not the shower, because he has a hole in his neck.
MISS BASS	*[Voice]* Got it. Don't worry, I will take care of him for you. Are you ready to go home?
BETTY	*[Voice]* Yes, but we must talk to Mrs. Cole before we leave.
MISS BASS	*(Turns to Val) [Sign]* Okay, Val, say goodbye to your parents.

Val walks away from Miss Bass and grabs his mother's pants. Miss Bass tries to grab him.

MISS BASS	*[Sign]* Come on, Val you need to stay here.
FALLON	*[Voice]* It is okay. Mrs. Cole will take care of everything. She will bring him back.
MISS BASS	*[Voice]* Sure, no problem. It was great meeting you two. Please be safe driving.

Val and his parents walk in the hallway to Mrs. Cole's office.

VAL	*[Sign]* Where are we going now?
FALLON	*[Sign]* To see Mrs. Cole and talk to her.
VAL	*[Sign]* She is a very nice lady.

BETTY   *[Sign]* Yes, she is. I'm glad you like her.

COLE   *[Voice]* Hello again. How is it going? Ready to go home?

FALLON   *[Voice]* Mrs. Cole, here is some information about Val's suction machine. Please give it to the nurse when you take him to the infirmary.

COLE   *[Voice]* Sure, no problem. I will be glad to give it to them. Why is Val with you?

BETTY   *[Voice]* He doesn't want us to go. We need to talk to you about something important before we leave.

COLE   *[Voice]* Sure. What is it?

BETTY   *[Voice]* Please take Val to the infirmary to be suctioned and brush his teeth after each meal. The machine will clean his trach. Please take care of our son.

FALLON   *[Voice]* We don't want him to go to the infirmary alone.

COLE   *[Voice]* Don't worry. I will be glad to take him there anytime.

BETTY   *[Voice]* Thanks so much, we don't want him to see us leave. How can we do that?

COLE   *[Voice to parents and sign to Val]* I have something for him to eat. *(Turns to Val)* Val, I have cookies and milk in my office. Do you want some?

VAL   *[Sign]* Yes, I want them.

BETTY   *[Voice]* Are the cookies soft?

COLE   *[Voice to Betty and sign to Val]* Yes, they are soft.

Let me take Val to my office. *(Turns to Val)* Come to my office. You can eat cookies here while I talk with your parents. Okay?

VAL   *[Sign]* Okay.

Mrs. Cole takes Val to her office and lets him use her desk to have cookies and milk.

COLE   *[Sign]* Get comfortable, we will be back. *(Cole closes the door of her office)*

COLE   *[Voice]* Everything is set up. You can leave and go home.

BETTY   *[Voice]* Are you sure Val will be alright?

COLE   *[Voice]* Don't worry, we will take care of him. Please be safe driving home.

BETTY   *[Voice]* We need to say goodbye to him and hug him.

FALLON   *[Voice]* It's okay, he will be alright. Let's go home. Thanks so much, Cole.

BETTY   *[Voice]* Cole, please take care of him for me; see you Friday.

COLE   *[Voice]* You're welcome, anytime. See you on Friday. Bye!

Fallon and Betty leave and go to the infirmary to deliver the suction machine and toothbrush, then they go home. Meanwhile, Val finishes eating only to find out his parents are missing.

VAL   *(Exits Cole's office) [Sign]* Cole, the cookies and milk were very good. Thanks so much. *(Hugs Cole)*

COLE   *[Sign]* Aww sweet. I am glad you liked them.

VAL   *(Looks around)* *[Sign]* Where is my mama and papa? Where did they go?

COLE   *[Sign]* Oh Val, I am afraid they left and went home.

VAL   *[Sign]* No, I need to go home with them! *(Runs outside)*

Cole runs and grabs Val's arm. They go back to Eagles Hall.

COLE   *[Sign]* Please listen to me. You will see them on Friday. We will take care of you.

VAL   *(Cries)* *[Sign]* I want Mama, and Papa, and Alan!

COLE   *(Holds Val)* *[Sign]* Please take it easy, don't worry, I will be here with you.

VAL   *(Cries)* *[Sign]* I want Mama, and Papa, and Alan!

COLE   *[Sign]* I know how you feel. You will see your family on Friday.

MISS BASS   *(Shows up)* *[Voice]* Cole, is Val okay?

COLE   *[Voice]* He will be alright soon. He is having a hard time accepting his parents' departure. He will get over it.

MISS BASS   *[Voice]* I understand. May I take him to the dorm?

COLE   *[Voice]* Not now. He will stay with me in my office and I will take him to the infirmary to be suctioned and brush his teeth. I will bring him back to the dorm. Okay?

MISS BASS   *[Voice]* I understand. Okay, I think Val is comfortable with you. See you later.

COLE   *[Voice to Miss Bass and sign to Val]]* Thanks, Miss

Bass. *(Hugs Val)* Oh dear, you will be alright.

VAL   *[Sign]* I want to be with you. *(He cries)*

COLE   *[Sign]* I am here with you.

Infirmary

Cole holds Val's hand as the go to the infirmary on the second floor of Woodard Hall.

COLE   *[Sign]* Val, here is the infirmary. This is where you will use your suction machine and your teeth will be cared for.

JEAN   *[Voice]* Hello Mrs. Cole, may I help you?

COLE   *[Voice]* Hello Jean. This is Val Melvin. He is here to clean his trach and brush his teeth. Here is an instruction paper about the suction machine.

JEAN   *[Voice to Cole and sign to Val]* Sure, his parents explained everything about him. Come on Val.

VAL   *(Tags Jean) [Sign]* What is your name?

JEAN   *[Sign]* Oh, my name is Jean Barnes. Don't be afraid, I will help you with your suctioning and your teeth brushing. Please come closer to the sink so I clean the trach.

Val moves closer to the sink and stands there while Jean cleans his trach and brushes his teeth.

COLE   *[Voice]* How is he doing?

JEAN   *[Voice]* He is doing fine. He knows what I'm doing for him. He is very good.

COLE   *[Sign to Val and voice to Jean]* Val, you are a very good boy. Let's go to the dorm and get ready for bed. *(Holds Val's hand)* Jean, thanks so much.

JEAN	*[Sign]* Okay, see you tomorrow.
VAL	*[Sign]* She is very nice. Is she the only nurse in the infirmary?
COLE	*[Sign]* No, you will meet another nurse tomorrow. Jean will train her how to clean your trach.

Mrs. Cole and Val go back to the boy's dorm as Miss Bass watches.

The Eagles Hall Dorm

COLE	*[Voice]* Hello Miss Bass. We are back from the infirmary, here is Val.
VAL	*[Sign]* Do I stay with her?
COLE	*[Sign]* Yes, she is your houseparent. She will take care of you.
MISS BASS	*[Sign]* Okay, Val it is time for a bath and then bed.
COLE	*[Voice]* I need to tell you something before Val's bath.
MISS BASS	*[Voice]* Sure, what is it?
COLE	*[Voice]* Please put him in the tub, not the shower. He is wearing the trach in his neck. Please be careful.
MISS BASS	*[Voice]* His mother told me that; what about his hair?
COLE	*[Voice]* Use the cup and put water on his hair; don't get too close to his neck, if you have a problem with that, please let me know.
MISS BASS	*[Voice]* Sure, I will take care of him.

COLE   *[Sign to Val and voice to Bass]* Val, please be very
                good for Miss Bass. Good night and I will see
                you tomorrow. *(Hugs Val)* Miss Bass, he is yours
                now. Good night.

VAL   *(Waves to Mrs. Cole) [Sign]* Good night Cole.

She leaves and goes to her office.

MISS BASS   *[Sign]* Please remove your clothes and go to the
                tub.

The Bathroom of the Eagles Hall Dorm

*Miss Bass has Val undress and cover with his towel. He goes to the tub as
the other boys stare at him. Miss Bass gets a cloth for him.*

VAL   *[Sign]* Miss Bass, I am ready.

MISS BASS   *[Sign]* Good boy, let me use the cloth to wash
                your body and pour water on your hair.

VAL   *[Sign]* Okay, be careful.

*Miss Bass washes Val's body with soap and washes his hair with shampoo,
she then dries him with the towel. Val puts on pajamas.*

The Bedroom of the Dorm

MISS BASS   *[Sign]* Here is your bed. Val, I will get a sheet,
                blanket, and pillow case for you. Please sit on the
                bed and I will be back soon.
VAL   *(Sits on his bed) [Sign]* Okay.

MISS BASS   *(Turns to the boys) [Sign]* Boys, please watch Val for
                me. I want all of you to be nice to him. He is
                new. I will be back soon. *(She leaves)*

The boys stare at him, but he ignores them.

BOY   *[Sign]* Who is the new boy?

BOY TWO   *[Sign]* His name is Val Melvin. Why does he have
                 a hole in his neck?

BOY   *[Sign]* I don't know. Just ask him.

BOY TWO   *(Turns to Val) [Sign]* What happened to your neck?

Val is silent and doesn't answer the question.

BOY TWO   *[Sign]* He ignored me; he's making me mad!

BOY   *[Sign]* He must be mute and dumb. Let's get him!

BOY TWO   *[Sign]* Your head is ugly!

Val cries and walks away from the boys.

BOY   *[Sign]* Wow, he cried like a baby.

*The boys are making fun of him, but he doesn't let them touch him. Miss
Bass shows up with the sheets and pillow case. She drops them and gets mad
at the boys.*

MISS BASS   *[Sign]* Stop! Boys go back to your beds. Stop
                  teasing Val and please leave him alone! I am
                  going to tell Mrs. Cole what happened! You are in
                  trouble.

MISS BASS   *(Holds Val) [Sign]* Are you alright, Val?

VAL   *(Cries and points to the boys) [Sign]* They called me
                  ugly. Please make them leave me alone.

MISS BASS   *[Sign]* Take it easy, I am here with you. *(She
                  continues to hold him and turns to the boys)* I am very
                  disappointed in both of you. You hurt his
                  feelings!

The Eagles Hall Dorm

Midnight, Cole comes to the dorm and finds Miss Bass, who is exhausted.

COLE   *[Voice]* Hello Miss Bass. I am here to check on
                Val. Is he alright?

MISS BASS   *[Voice]* He's not good, the boys stared at the hole
                in his neck and made fun of him. It was tough on
                him, I moved him to another bed where nobody
                will bother him. He is asleep now. I feel bad for
                him.

COLE   *[Voice]* That's mean. It makes me mad. I need to
                see him now, I am concerned about him.

MISS BASS   *[Voice]* Sure, come with me.

COLE   *[Voice]* Where is Val?

MISS BASS   *(Points to Val, sleeping in the bed) [Voice]* Here he is.

COLE   *(Goes to the bed and pats his head) [Voice]* All of the
                boys teased him?

MISS BASS   *[Voice]* I am afraid so. How can we get them to be
                nice to him?

COLE   *[Voice]* Don't worry, I will explain everything
                about Val to them after school tomorrow. Is it
                okay with you if Val stays with me for breakfast?

MISS BASS   *[Voice]* Yes, he is comfortable with you. I don't
                think he likes me.

COLE   *[Voice]* Did he say something bad to you?

MISS BASS   *[Voice]* No, he was very nice to me until the boys
                teased him. He kept screaming and kicking. He is
                hurt.

COLE   *[Voice]* I understand, you tried your best. I will
                talk to him, okay?

MISS BASS   *[Voice]* Okay.

| COLE | *[Voice]* Thanks for telling me what happened. Please take him to my office tomorrow morning. Good night. |
| MISS BASS | *[Voice]* Sure, good night Cole. |

Scene Two: The First Day of School

In the morning Miss Bass gets Val dressed and ties his shoes. She tries to brush his hair, but Val doesn't let her. The boys keep staring at him and they say more mean things. Miss Bass takes Val to Mrs. Cole's office.

MISS BASS	*[Voice]* Good morning Cole, here is Val. He is still having a hard time with the boys.
COLE	*(Looks at Val)* *[Voice]* Why is his hair messy?
MISS BASS	*[Voice]* He wouldn't let me brush it. You are the only one he trusts to do it. Here is his brush. I will let him stay with you during breakfast.
COLE	*[Voice]* Okay, thanks, I will do that and I will talk to him. See you later.
MISS BASS	*[Voice to Cole and sign to Val]* Thanks Cole. See you later, Val. *(She leaves)*
COLE	*[Sign]* Good morning Val. Please let me brush your hair; breakfast is almost ready.
VAL	*[Sign]* Okay.
COLE	*(Brushes his hair)* *[Sign]* Good boy. Why don't you like Miss Bass? She is very sweet.
VAL	*[Sign]* I like her, but I don't like the boys. They call me ugly.
COLE	*[Sign]* I understand what you mean. She is upset about the boys teasing you. She doesn't want to

see you hurt. Please tell her you are sorry and be
nice to her.

VAL   *[Sign]* Okay, I am very sorry.

COLE   *[Sign]* You can tell her after breakfast. Do you
               like to eat Rice Krispies?

VAL   *[Sign]* Yes, I am hungry.

COLE   *[Sign]* I know you are. Let's go to the lunchroom
               for breakfast, and please stay with me.

The Lunchroom

In the lunchroom, Cole and Val sit together and eat eggs, grits, and Rice Krispies.

COLE   *[Sign]* Val, eat your breakfast please.

VAL   *[Sign]* Okay, but why are the girls staring at me? Is
               it the hole in my neck?

COLE   *[Sign]* Ignore them. I will explain everything to
               them. Please don't worry.

VAL   *[Sign]* Okay. Who will take me to the infirmary?

COLE   *[Sign]* Me, and you will meet another nurse today.
               Eat your breakfast before it is time to go.

After they finish breakfast, they go to the infirmary for suctioning and teeth brushing.

They see Miss Bass in the infirmary and she agrees to escort Val into the hallway.

The middle of Eagles Hall

MISS BASS   *[Sign]* It is time to go to class, come with me.

VAL	*[Sign]* Okay. I am so sorry I was mean to you. I know you are trying to help me.
MISS BASS	*[Sign]* It is okay, you are a good boy.
VAL	*(Hugs Miss Bass) [Sign]* Okay, see you later.
MISS BASS	*(Pats his head) [Sign]* Aww sweet. Have fun at school.
SIMMONS	*[Sign]* Good morning Val! I am going to take you to your classroom. I hope you enjoy it.

Humphrey's Classroom

Simmons escorts Val to the classroom and Humphrey greets them. The other students stare at him.

SIMMONS	*[Voice]* Good morning, Mrs. Humphrey.
HUMPHREY	*[Sign]* Good morning, Simmons, good morning, Val. Welcome to our classroom!
VAL	*(Waves at her) [Sign]* Good morning, Mrs. Humphrey.
SIMMONS	*[Voice to Humphrey and sign to Val]* He is shy and quiet. He had a hard time yesterday because the kids kept staring at him. *(Turns to Val)* Please be good to Humphrey.
VAL	*[Sign]* Okay.
SIMMONS	*[Voice]* Let me know if you have any problems with Val. Have a good day.
HUMPHREY	*[Voice to Simmons and sign to Val]* Okay. *(Turns to Val)* Val, please take a seat next to Traci. Let me put your hearing aid on.

Humphrey puts Val's haring aid on his head.

HUMPHREY   *[Sign]* Are you comfortable?

Val nods and sits next to Traci.

TRACI   *[Sign]* I am not sure if I like him or not. He is different.

STEPHEN   *[Sign]* He looks like an ugly duckling.

HUMPHREY   *[Sign]* Stephen! Stop teasing him, please be nice to him.

STEPHEN   *[Sign]* Okay.

HUMPHREY   *[Sign]* Kids, I want all of you to be nice to Val, he is new here. Tell him who you are.

CAROLINA   *[Sign]* My name is Carolina Enriquez.

CASSANDRA   *[Sign]* My name is Cassandra Porter.

CINDY   *[Sign]* My name is Cindy Williams.

CORIE   *[Sign]* My name is Corie Jackson.

JUNIOR   *[Sign]* My name is Junior Harrison.

KATHY   *[Sign]* My name is Kathy Yott.

MATTHEW   *[Sign]* My name is Matthew Halstead.

STEPHEN   *[Sign]* My name is Stephen Phillips.

TRACI   *[Sign]* My name is Traci Baines.

HUMPHREY   *[Sign]* Thanks so much! *(Turns to Val)* Tell us about yourself. Please don't be shy.

VAL   *[Sign]* Hello, my name is Val Melvin. I am seven years old and live in New Bern.

HUMPHREY   *[Sign]* Good boy, how many siblings do you have?

VAL   *[Sign]* I have one brother, his name is Alan and he
             is ten years old.

HUMPHREY   *[Sign]* Thanks, any questions about Val?

STEPHEN   *(Raises his hand)* *[Sign]* How did he get a hole in his
             neck?

Val gets mad, goes to the restroom, and locks the door.

HUMPHREY   *[Sign]* Oh no! *(Turns to Stephen)* Stephen! It is not
             very nice to ask a question like that. Let me get
             him.

Humphrey gets a key and unlocks the door.

STEPHEN   *[Sign]* I am so sorry. I just asked a question, that's
             all.

HUMPHREY   *(Pulls Val by the hand)* *[Sign]* Come on Val, please
             sit down. Thanks, do you have a sign name?

VAL   *[Sign]* No, fingerspell: V A L.

HUMPHREY   *[Sign]* Okay. Kids, please pay attention to me. I
             am going to begin to teach a new lesson: spelling.
             Ready?

TRACI   *(Raises her hand)* *[Sign]* Mrs. Humphrey?

HUMPHREY   *[Sign]* Yes?

TRACI   *[Sign]* Can I move to sit next to Carolina, please?

HUMPHREY   *[Sign]* Why?

TRACI   *[Sign]* I don't like Val. His head is ugly.

Val cries and goes back to the restroom.

HUMPHREY   *[Sign]* You hurt his feelings. You can move to sit
             next to Carolina if you want. I am disappointed in

all you. *(Turns to Val)* Please come on and sit down. I am here with you.

Traci moves next to Carolina as Humphrey opens the restroom door and pulls Val back to his seat.

VAL   *[Sign]* I don't think they like me.

HUMPHREY   *[Sign]* I know. I will explain everything to them and make them be very nice. Ignore them if they say bad things about you. Okay?

VAL   *[Sign]* Okay.

HUMPHREY   *[Sign]* Matthew, why did you move closer to Kathy? Do you like her?

MATTHEW   *[Sign]* I want to be closer to her. I am more comfortable here.

KATHY   *[Sign]* Not true. I know you want to move far away from Val.

Val gets up.

HUMPHREY   *[Sign]* Val, please sit down. *(Turns to the kids)* I want all of you to be nice to him. He has a birth defect and can't help that he is different.

CINDY   *[Sign]* What is a birth defect?

HUMPHREY   *[Sign]* It means that he was born a little different than you.

CINDY   *[Sign]* Ew! I am not going to touch him. Please get him away from us!

CASSANDRA   *[Sign]* Can you move him to the other classroom?

CORIE   *[Sign]* We are so sorry, but we don't want him here. Get him out of the classroom!

Val cries and runs away from the classroom.

HUMPHREY *[Sign]* Val don't do that! *(Turns to the kids)* Please stay here, all of you are in trouble. I am going to get him now. *(She leaves)*

STEPHEN *[Sign]* I think he is going to the asylum soon.

The kids laugh.

Miss Simmons comes out of her office and sees Val running in the hallway.

SIMMONS *[Sign]* Val! Stop running! You are supposed to be with Mrs. Humphrey!

Val ignores her and runs outside.

Mrs. Cole and Mrs. Humphrey enter the hallway. They see Val run outside.

COLE *[Voice]* Simmons, what happened?

SIMMONS *[Voice]* I don't know. Humphrey, what's wrong with him? He is acting crazy. We need to find him before he gets hurt or lost.

HUMPHREY *[Voice]* The students hurt his feelings and told him they don't like him. It broke my heart.

COLE *[Voice]* We will talk about it later. Let's find him now.

They go outside and begin searching for Val.

SIMMONS *[Voice]* He is very good at hiding from us. Where is he?

COLE *(Holds Val's hand) [Voice]* I found him in the bush. He is fine, but crying a lot.

SIMMONS *[Voice]* Good job, Cole! I am going to take him to my office and teach him a lesson.

HUMPHREY   *[Voice]* No! The students are responsible for this. I will punish them.

SIMMONS   *[Voice]* Okay, I will straighten them out. Humphrey, please take him back to the classroom now.

VAL   *(Turns to Cole) [Sign]* I want to stay with you. I don't want to stay with Mrs. Humphrey, the kids don't like me.

COLE   *[Sign to Val and voice to Simmons]* Take it easy, she is your teacher. She will take care of everything. *(Turns to Simmons)* What are we going to do with him if he refuses to go?

SIMMONS   *[Voice]* Well, I better go to my office to get the belt now.

HUMPHREY   *[Voice]* Are you going to spank him?

SIMMONS   *[Voice]* Wait and see; I will be right back. *(She leaves and goes to her office)*

COLE   *(Turns to Val) [Sign]* Listen to me. I want you to be good for Mrs. Humphrey, she will take care of you.

VAL   *[Sign]* But the kids don't like me.

COLE   *[Sign]* I know, but ignore what they say about you. Please tell Mrs. Humphrey you are sorry. You hurt her feelings.

VAL   *[Sign]* Okay. *(Turns to Humphrey)* I am very sorry.

HUMPHREY   *[Sign]* Thanks, come back to the classroom with me.

SIMMONS   *[Voice]* I am back. Here is the belt.

COLE   *[Voice]* What are you going to do with the belt, spank him?

SIMMONS   *[Voice]* Watch. *(She ties the belt around Val's arm and gives it to Humphrey)* You can pull it to take Val to the classroom.

HUMPHREY   *[Sign and voice]* That's crazy! He is not a dog!

COLE   *[Sign and voice]* Well, *(Turns to Val)* please behave yourself for Humphrey.

VAL   *[Sign]* Okay. I don't like Simmons.

SIMMONS   *(Turns to Val) [Sign]* What did you say?

VAL   *[Sign]* Nothing.

SIMMONS   *[Sign]* Please tell me the truth or I will spank you.

VAL   *(Nervously) [Sign]* I don't like you.

SIMMONS   *[Voice and sign]* That's it! *(Spanks Val's butt and he cries)* Humphrey, let's go back to the classroom so I can speak with your students.

HUMPHREY   *(Sighs) [Sign]* Val come with me.

Humphrey pulls Val and they go back to the classroom. Cole goes back to her office.

SIMMONS   *[Sign]* Kids, I am here to tell you something. It is not nice to say bad things about Val. I want you to apologize to him for being mean or I will spank all of you with the ruler.

STEPHEN   *[Sign]* We are not mean to him. We just don't like him at all.

SIMMONS   *[Sign]* Well, is it true?

JUNIOR   *[Sign]* Stephen! You made Miss Simmons mad at us.

SIMMONS   *[Sign]* Junior, don't say anything. Please tell me the truth now.

The kids are silent.

SIMMONS   *[Sign]* That's it. Give me your hands. *(She spanks their hands with a ruler as Humphrey and Val look on)* You better learn your lesson.

Val laughs at his classmates.

Simmons turns to face Val.

SIMMONS   *[Sign]* What are you laughing at?

VAL   *[Sign]* Nothing.

SIMMONS   *[Sign]* I know you laughed at your classmates. Please go to the hallway now.

Val goes to the hallway as Humphrey watches.

HUMPHREY   *[Voice]* Simmons, why did you send him to the hallway?

SIMMONS   *[Voice]* Wait and see. Please stay here. I will be back.

She leaves and meets Val in the hallway.

SIMMONS   *[Sign]* Val, please give your hands to me.

VAL   *(Puts his hands out)* *[Sign]* Please don't do that to me.

Simmons spanks Val's hands with the ruler as Val cries.

SIMMONS   *[Sign]* You better have learned your lesson; go back to the classroom now.

VAL	*[Sign]* Okay.
SIMMONS	*[Voice]* Here he is. Please let me know if something happens again.

She leaves.

HUMPHREY	*[Voice to Simmons and sign to Val]* Okay, *(Turns to Val)* are you alright?
VAL	*[Sign]* My hands are hurt! She is mean!
HUMPHREY	*[Sign]* Take it easy. I am here with you. Let's have class.

In the lunchroom, Humphrey and the kids are at the table. Val sits next to Humphrey because nobody else wants to sit next to him. Val refuses to eat his lunch.

HUMPHREY	*[Sign]* Val, eat your lunch; it is good.
VAL	*(Tastes greens) [Sign]* I don't like it. It is terrible. *(Drinks milk)*
TRACI	*[Sign]* Humphrey, why does he keep drinking milk and not eating anything?
HUMPHREY	*[Sign]* Please let me handle this. *(Turns to Val)* Stop drinking milk, I want you to eat your lunch. You will be starving later.
VAL	*[Sign]* I am not hungry. I don't want it.
HUMPHREY	*[Sign]* Why do you keep drinking milk?
VAL	*[Sign]* I like it.
HUMPHREY	*[Sign]* Do you know where milk comes from?

VAL	*[Sign]* I don't know.
HUMPHREY	*[Sign]* It comes from a cow. They make milk.
VAL	*[Sign]* Do they make chocolate milk?
HUMPHREY	*[Sign]* No, white milk is mixed with chocolate syrup.

Simmons shows up to check on how Val is doing.

SIMMONS	*[Voice]* Humphrey, has Val eaten lunch yet?
HUMPHREY	*[Voice]* A little, he is mostly drinking milk, though.
SIMMONS	*(Sighs) [Voice]* It is time for him to go to the infirmary.
HUMPHREY	*[Voice]* He goes there alone?
SIMMONS	*[Voice]* No, he needs someone to go with him.
HUMPHREY	*[Sign]* Okay, *(Turns to her students)* do you want to take Val to the infirmary?

The students refuse to answer her question.

HUMPHREY	*(Sighs) [Sign]* I guess I have to take him to the infirmary. Who will watch the kids?
SIMMONS	*[Voice]* I will. Here is the belt to pull Val to the infirmary.
HUMPHREY	*[Voice]* Oh no, I don't want his arm tied like a dog.
SIMMONS	*(Ties the belt around Val's arm) [Voice]* Okay, take him to the infirmary.
HUMPHREY	*[Sign]* Come on, Val.
VAL	*[Sign]* I am not a dog!

HUMPHREY   *[Sign]* I know. I don't like how she treats you;
             please obey me.

VAL   *[Sign]* Okay.

*Mrs. Humphrey holds the belt and takes Val to the infirmary. Jean Barnes
is shocked to see to see this.*

JEAN   *(Surprised) [Voice]* Hello. Why are you doing this to
             Val? Did you do this?

HUMPHREY   *[Voice]* I didn't do this. Simmons tied it around
             his arm to make sure Val doesn't run away from
             me.

JEAN   *[Voice to Humphrey and sign to Val]* That's mean.
             Let me bring Val to the doctor's exam room.
             Come on, Val.

HUMPHREY   *[Voice]* Do you mind if I watch you suction Val? I
             would like to learn how.

JEAN   *[Voice]* Sure, you can.

Jean cleans Val's trach and brushes his teeth as Mrs. Humphrey looks on.

*Humphrey pulls the belt to take Val back to Eagles Hall. They step into the
hallway.*

VAL   *[Sign]* Mrs. Humphrey?

HUMPHREY   *[Sign]* Yes, Val?

VAL   *[Sign]* Can you remove the belt from my arm? It is
             rough. It hurts me!

HUMPHREY   *[Sign]* What about Miss Simmons? She will get
             mad if the belt is not around your arm.

VAL   *[Sign]* But you don't like it.

HUMPHREY   *[Sign]* You are right, but promise you won't run away from me?

VAL   *[Sign]* I won't.

HUMPHREY   *(Unties the belt)* *[Sign]* Okay. Come with me to the classroom.

VAL   *(Smiles)* *[Sign]* Thanks, Mrs. Humphrey.

Humphrey goes to Mrs. Cole's office.

COLE   *[Voice]* Good afternoon Mrs. Humphrey. Where did you come from?

HUMPHREY   *[Voice]* Good afternoon! I just took Val to the infirmary.

COLE   *(Confused)* *[Voice]* I don't see him. Where is he?

HUMPHREY   *[Voice]* He is here with me. *(Looks around)* Oh no, he did it again!

COLE   *[Voice]* Well, would you like me to help you find him?

HUMPHREY   *[Voice]* No thanks. I think he is in the girls' dorm hallway. I am going to find him.

Humphrey goes to the girl's dorm and looks around.

VAL   *[Sign]* Hello Mrs. Humphrey. I am here.

HUMPHREY   *[Sign]* Where have you been? You scared me!

VAL   *[Sign]* I had to pee.

HUMPHREY   *[Sign]* You could have told me that. You are in trouble Val!

VAL   *[Sign]* Are you mad?

HUMPHREY	*(Spanks Val's hand) [Sign]* Yes, you scared me. I am going to tie the belt around your arm. *(She ties the belt around his arm)*
VAL	*(Cries) [Sign]* Don't do that. I just went to the restroom, that's all.
HUMPHREY	*[Sign]* Please take it easy. Simmons is at our classroom. I don't want her to find out, okay?
VAL	*[Sign]* Okay. I don't like it.
HUMHPREY	*[Sign]* I will untie it when Simmons leaves. Please be patient.

Eagles Hall Playground

Humphrey and the class are outside. The kids are on the merry-go-round, but Val is on the swing. Humphrey walks over to him.

HUMPHREY	*[Sign]* Val, why don't you play with your classmates?
VAL	*[Sign]* They won't let me play with them.
HUMPHREY	*[Sign]* Okay, I will talk to them.

Humphrey walks over to her students.

HUMPHREY	*[Sign]* Kids, why don't you let Val play with all of you?
TRACI	*[Sign]* He is very different from us.
HUMPHREY	*[Sign]* He is not that different, he is deaf like all of you.
STEPHEN	*[Sign]* I know, but he is the only one who has a hole in his neck. He is different from us.
HUMPHREY	*[Sign]* Kids, I am disappointed in all of you for

not listening to me about Val.

CAROLINA   *[Sign]* Look at Val, he is on the swing. It looks like he is having lots of fun.

HUMPHREY   *(Looks at Val) [Sign]* See? He can do everything you do.

CINDY   *[Sign]* Look at him. The swing is getting higher. You need to watch him.

HUMPHREY   *(Screams and runs to Val) [Sign]* No! No! STOP!

Val falls off the swing.

HUMPHREY   *[Sign]* Are you alright Val?

VAL   *[Sign]* That was fun. I like it.

HUMPHREY   [Sign] Don't swing too high. It is time to go to the classroom.

After school the class is dismissed. The kids go to the dorm and Humphrey gets ready to go home.

The Middle of Eagles Hall

SIMMONS   *[Voice]* Hello Humphrey. How was your first day?

HUMPHREY   *[Voice]* Not good.

SIMMONS   *[Voice]* Because of Val?

HUMPHREY   *[Voice]* Right. He didn't do anything because the kids kept avoiding him. I had a hard time making them be nice to him.

SIMMONS   *[Voice]* I know what you mean. I am not sure if we should keep Val or not. He has a hard time listening to what we tell him to do.

HUMPHREY   *[Voice]* Okay. Are you going to call his parents to tell them what happened today? They will be heartbroken.

SIMMONS   *[Voice]* I'd rather tell them in person when they come here. Wait a minute, Val's father works at Carolina Power and Light.

HUMPHREY   *[Voice]* That's right. He is a Methodist pastor too.

SIMMONS   *[Voice]* Oh, Val doesn't look like he is a pastor's son. He is different from his father.

HUMPHREY   *[Voice]* He was born with a birth defect. We don't know what to do with him.

COLE   *[Voice]* Good afternoon. I got a call from Mrs. Melvin.

HUMPHREY   *[Voice]* Good. How is she doing? Did you tell her what happened today?

COLE   *[Voice]* I lied to her and told her everything went well. I don't want to upset her, but I feel bad about lying. I know Mr. Melvin is a pastor.

SIMMONS   *[Voice]* I know what you mean. You don't need to tell her about today. I will tell her on Friday when she comes to pick Val up.

HUMPHREY   *[Voice]* Wait a minute. Are you going to tell her about the kids treating him badly?

SIMMONS   *[Voice]* No, why?

HUMPHREY   *[Voice]* I am so sorry. I hope you won't tell her about that.

SIMMONS   *[Voice]* It is okay. Don't worry, everything will be alright with Val soon.

HUMPHREY	*[Voice]* Val might tell them about the kids.
SIMMONS	*[Voice]* What can we do?
COLE	*[Voice]* Got it!
HUMPHREY	*[Voice]* What?
COLE	*[Voice]* I will keep Val from telling his parents about the kids. I will give him cake and milk if he won't tell his parents.
HUMPHREY	*[Voice]* Good idea! When would you tell Val not to tell them?
COLE	*[Voice]* Thursday night.

Scene Three: Val Has a Rough Day

Eagles Hall Playground

The kids play outside. Val looks for someone to play with him, but they keep avoiding him.

VAL	*[Sign]* Hello, may I play with you?
STEPHEN	*[Sign]* No thanks. I want you to go away.
VAL	*[Sign]* I want to be your friend.
STEPHEN	*[Sign]* I know, but we don't want to be your friends. You are very different from us.
VAL	*[Sign]* Why am I different?
STEPHEN	You have a hole in your neck but we don't. That's why. We want you to leave us alone.
VAL	*[Sign]* I feel lonely.

STEPHEN	*[Sign]* Well, play with your invisible friend.
VAL	*[Sign]* I guess so. *(He leaves)*
JUNIOR	*[Sign]* Stephen, you hurt his feelings.
STEPHEN	*[Sign]* Who cares? We need to get rid of him.
MATTHEW	*[Sign]* How?
STEPHEN	*[Sign]* His parents will find out nobody likes him and then they will pull him from the school.
JUNIOR	*[Sign]* Wait and see.
STEPHEN	*[Sign]* Huh? You like him.
JUNIOR	*[Sign]* Not sure. I need to see what his parents look like.
STEPHEN	*[Sign]* His parents are ugly like him.
JUNIOR	*[Sign]* What if his mother is beautiful?

Stephen says nothing and plays ball with the boys. Junior feels very bad for Val as he watches him go into the dorm.

Miss Bass looks for Val in the dorm and finds him lying on his bed. Val holds his sock monkey.

The Eagles Hall Dorm bedroom

MISS BASS	*[Sign]* Val, are you alright?
VAL	*[Sign]* No. I am very sad because nobody likes me.
MISS BASS	*[Sign]* I'm sorry, what do you want me to do?
VAL	*[Sign]* Can you help me make friends? I am lonely.

MISS BASS	*[Sign]* Oh dear, I know how you feel. I will ask them if they want to play with you.
VAL	*[Sign]* Who?
MISS BASS	*[Sign]* Wait and see. Come with me. You will like them.
VAL	*[Sign]* Where are we going?
MISS BASS	*[Sign]* To the girls' dorm, they might like you.

The Girls' TV room

They go to the girls' dorm and find the girls in the TV room. Bass talks to their houseparent.

MISS BASS	*[Sign]* Hello girls, I would like all of you to meet this boy. His name is Val Melvin. He would like to make friends with all of you.
CAROLINA	*[Sign]* I know him. He is my classmate, but I don't want to be his friend. Please get him out of here.
CINDY	*[Sign]* No way. Go away. Take him back to the boys' dorm.
MISS BASS	*[Sign]* But he has hard time making friends with the boys.
CINDY	*[Sign]* Why doesn't he make friends with the adults like you?
MISS BASS	*[Sign]* Sigh, I guess we should go now.
VAL	*[Sign]* They don't like me! I want to go home!
CASSANDRA	*[Sign]* Why don't you quit school and stay home with your parents?
GIRLS'	*[Voice]* Sorry, Miss Bass. I tried to make them

HOUSEPARENT	be nice to him, but they won't listen to me. I am sorry.
MISS BASS	*[Voice and sign]* It is okay, thanks. *(Turns to Val)* Let's go back to our dorm. *(They leave)*

That night, the boys watch TV, but Val sits alone in the hallways as Miss Bass looks on. Miss Bass helps Val get ready for bed. She is in tears and goes to Mrs. Cole's office.

Cole's Office

COLE	*[Voice]* Hello Bass. You look very disappointed. Is everything okay with Val?
MISS BASS	*[Voice]* Not good. I tried to help him make friends with the children, but they keep avoiding him. I feel sorry for him.
COLE	*[Voice]* Too bad. I am disappointed they didn't listen to me about Val. I can't tell his parents what happened.
MISS BASS	*[Voice]* I know what you mean. They will be heartbroken. If they find out, will they pull Val out?
COLE	*[Voice]* No way! I don't want to upset them. He is a sweet boy. I don't want to lose him. How did you two get along?
MISS BASS	*[Voice]* He seems to trust me when I help him to dress. He thinks I am very sweet. He is always with me since the boys keep avoiding him.
COLE	*[Voice]* I am glad that you two are getting along. What about making friends with the girls?

MISS BASS	*[Voice]* Well, they did the same thing the boys did.
COLE	*[Voice]* I need to talk to Miss Simmons about what happened. We will work on making everyone like Val.
MISS BASS	*[Voice]* I hope it will work out. I better go now because I need to check on the boys. I will talk to you later. Good night.
COLE	*[Voice]* Thanks so much. Good night, I am glad that you and Val are getting along well.
MISS BASS	*[Voice]* I almost forgot, will you eat breakfast with Val tomorrow morning?
COLE	*[Voice]* Excuse me? I thought you two got along well. What went wrong?
MISS BASS	*[Voice]* The boys asked me if Val would eat breakfast with you. They are uncomfortable with him.
COLE	*(Gets mad) [Voice]* Aw, that's rude. I will punish them tomorrow.

The next morning Humphrey arrives to school late and finds Mrs. Cole in her office. She is in a bad mood.

Eagles Hall Foyer

HUMPHREY	*[Voice]* Good morning Cole. I am so sorry I am late for school. One of my sons went to school late. How is Val doing?
COLE	*[Voice]* Good morning Humphrey, Val is alright, but I am not in a mood to talk. Thanks.

HUMPHREY   *[Voice]* I understand, I better leave you alone.

Middle of Eagles Hall

SIMMONS   *[Voice]* Good morning Humphrey. I
                  understand why you are late for school. I am
                  glad you called me. Your class is waiting for
                  you.

HUMPHREY   *[Voice]* Thanks! Cole looks very upset, what's
                  wrong?

SIMMONS   *[Voice]* She had a hard time with the children
                  because they didn't listen to her about Val.
                  Cole asked us to have a meeting with her
                  about him.

HUMPHREY   *[Voice]* What time is the meeting?

SIMMONS   *[Voice]* I will let you know later. Your students
                  are waiting for you.

HUMPHREY   *[Voice]* Okay, I hope you have a chance to
                  keep Val in school.

SIMMONS   *[Voice]* We will have to wait and see.

Humphrey's classroom

*Humphrey goes to the classroom and finds Val sitting at his desk while the
other students sit at the class table.*

HUMPHREY   *[Sign]* Kids, why is Val sitting at his desk
                  alone?

TRACI   *[Sign]* He wants to sit alone. That's all.

HUMPHREY   *[Sign]* Well, is it true?

The students nod.

HUMPHREY	*[Sign]* Okay. I am going to ask him why.
TRACI	*[Sign]* You don't believe us? Do you?
HUMPHREY	*[Sign]* Wait and find out. *(Turns to Val)* Val, why are you sitting at your desk alone?
VAL	*[Sign]* They don't want me to sit with them so I sat here.
STEPHEN	*(Gets up) [Sign]* Wrong! He lied. You better believe us.
HUMPHREY	*[Sign]* Do you know Val's father is a pastor?

The students gasp.

HUMPHREY	*[Sign]* Please tell me the truth now.
JUNIOR	*[Sign]* Humphrey, Val is right.
STEPHEN	*[Sign]* Junior! Why did you do that?
JUNIOR	*[Sign]* His father is a pastor. I have to be honest with Humphrey. I am so sorry I did that to Val.
HUMPHREY	*[Sign]* Junior, you did the right thing. You are all punished except Junior.
STEPHEN	*[Sign]* Thanks so much Junior!

Teacher's lounge

Simmons, Humphrey, and Cole are in the Teacher's lounge for a meeting about Val. Mrs. Cole tells them she wants to keep Val in school.

COLE	*[Voice]* I am so sorry about this morning. I need to discuss the children with you. They didn't listen to me about Val. That's why I was upset.

SIMMONS	*[Voice]* It is hard to find a friend for Val. They see he is different; they think he might be retarded.
COLE	*[Voice]* Wrong! The hole in his neck doesn't mean he is retarded. His parents want him to learn like the other children. He is special.
HUMPHREY	*[Voice]* I agree with Cole. He needs to learn everything. That's what his parents want him to do. He finally found a friend.
COLE AND SIMMONS	*[Voice]* Who?
HUMPHREY	*[Voice]* It is Junior Harrison. He became friends with Val when I told my students that his father is a pastor. I gave him a star and I punished the others.
SIMMONS	*[Voice]* Wow! That's clever. I am glad to hear, but you need to make the others be friends with Val.
COLE	*[Voice]* It is hard to get the kids to trust him. They don't like him. I need someone to change their mind.
HUMPHREY	*[Voice]* Cole, you have a meeting with Val tonight. What is it about?
COLE	*[Voice]* I have to talk to Val and ask him to keep a secret from his parents about the children.
SIMMONS	*[Voice]* The meeting is over, we will have to keep thinking of a solution. I hope the problem will be solved.
HUMPHREY	*[Voice]* Amen!

DAWSON	*(Shows up)* *[Voice]* Humphrey, I need to tell you something; it is about Val. You won't like it.
HUMPHREY	*[Voice]* Really? What is it?
DAWSON	*[Voice]* I wouldn't let him come in until you see him.
HUMPHREY	*[Voice]* Why didn't you let him come in?
DAWSON	*[Voice]* Come and see; follow me.
HUMPHREY	*[Voice]* Cole, thanks for the meeting. Talk to you later.

Dawson and Humphrey go to the playground.

HUMPHREY	*[Voice]* I don't understand, what are you talking about?
DAWSON	*[Voice]* You will find out when you see him.
HUMPHREY	*[Voice]* What's wrong with him?

Dawson and Humphrey walk outside and find Val in the mud.

DAWSON	*[Voice]* Here he is.
HUMPHREY	*(Gets upset)* *[Sign]* Val, why are you in the mud?
VAL	*(Looks at Humphrey)* *[Sign]* I am so sorry. I accidentally fell down.
HUMPHREY	*[Sign]* Well, it is time for your bath!
VAL	*(Looks sad)* *[Sign]* Am I bad?
HUMPHREY	*[Sign]* Yes, you are bad. You don't need to play in the mud again. I don't like it.
VAL	*[Sign]* Humphrey, I am sorry.

Humphrey pulls Val from the mud and gets him undressed. She puts him in the tub and washes his body and hair. Humphrey tells Val not to play in the mud again. Val nods in agreement.

Cole's Office

That night Mrs. Cole invites Val to go to her office. He is wearing pajamas and a robe.

VAL	*[Sign]* Hello Cole, Miss Bass told me you need to talk to me now. I am so sorry about the mud.
COLE	*[Sign]* It is okay, but that's not it. Please sit down.
VAL	*(Smiles) [Sign]* Okay. I like this couch better than the one in the TV room.
COLE	*[Sign]* I am glad you like it. Please listen to me. I would like you to keep a secret.
VAL	*[Sign]* What does secret mean?
COLE	*[Sign]* Oh! You don't know what it is? It is something you don't want another person to know. Please don't tell your parents and Alan about what happened.
VAL	*[Sign]* Okay. What is our secret?
COLE	*[Sign]* I am glad you asked me that. I want you to tell your parents that you like the school and are making friends.
VAL	*[Sign]* You want to me to lie to them? Papa won't like it.
COLE	*[Sign]* I know what you mean. I don't want you to leave school, I would miss you. *(In tears)* I want you to stay longer because I love you.

VAL   *(Smiles) [Sign]* Aw, I love you too.

Scene Four: The Letter about Val's Birth

The next day, Humphrey has a hard time with Val, but still feels bad for him. She wonders how to get Val to trust her. Humphrey knows Cole is the only one Val trusts. She decides to see Cole.

Cole's Office

HUMPHREY   *[Voice]* Hello Cole. I need to ask you questions about Val.

COLE   *[Voice]* Sure, what is it?

HUMPHREY   *[Voice]* I need to know everything about him, so I can get him to trust me.

COLE   *[Voice]* What do you want to know about him?

HUMPHREY   *[Voice]* Like his birth and how he got the hole in his neck.

COLE   *[Voice]* I understand. I suggest you ask his parents, but Mrs. Melvin would rather write a letter instead of talking on the phone about him.

HUMPHREY   *[Voice]* Sure, I will call her and ask her to write me a letter. I am anxious.

COLE   *[Voice]* I understand, it looks like you care about him.

HUMPHREY   *[Voice]* I do. I am having a hard time with him. He keeps avoiding me; I have decided to get to know him better.

COLE   *[Voice]* Okay, well, good luck. I want the two
                   of you to get along well. Please let me know
                   when you two get closer.

HUMPHREY   *[Voice]* Sure, thanks. Have a good evening.
                   Please keep Val out of trouble.

One week later Humphrey is home and tired from school. She sits on the
couch to rest and her husband, CW, brings letters to her.

CW   *[Voice]* Hello Mary Sue, you look frustrated.
                   Did Val give you a hard time?

HUMPHREY   *[Voice]* No, I tried to make my students be
                   nice to him, but they keep avoiding him. He
                   cries a lot because he is upset nobody likes
                   him.

CW   *[Voice]* Oh, sorry. You got mail today.

HUMPHREY   *[Voice]* Really?

CW   *[Voice]* Yes. The letter is from Mrs. Melvin.
                   (CW gives the letter to his wife)

HUMPHREY   *[Voice]* Great! I am looking forward to
                   reading it, but I am too nervous to read.

CW   *[Voice]* Why?

HUMPHREY   *[Voice]* I asked Mrs. Melvin to write a letter
                   to me about his birth and the hole in his
                   neck.

CW   *[Voice]* Oh, do you want me to be with you
                   when you read the letter?

HUMPHREY   *[Voice]* Well, I will tell you about it after
                   reading it.

CW	*[Voice]* Okay, if you need me, I will be in the backyard.
HUMPHREY	*[Voice]* Okay thanks, honey.
CW	*[Voice]* I love you.
HUMPHREY	*(Kisses her husband) [Voice]* Love you too.

CW goes outside to clean the truck while Humphrey looks at the envelope and opens it. She reads the letter about Val's birth and is in tears by the end.

During the night, CW and Humphrey are in bed, but Humphrey is unable to sleep because she can't stop thinking about Val. CW wakes up and realizes his wife is still awake.

CW	*[Voice]* Mary Sue, you okay?
HUMPHREY	*[Voice]* Yes, but I can't sleep. I can't stop thinking about Val.
CW	*[Voice]* Oh dear. It is the letter isn't it?
HUMPHREY	*[Voice]* That's right. It is about his birth. He spent two months in Duke Hospital after his birth.
CW	*[Voice]* Wow! Why did he stay there so long?
HUMPHREY	*[Voice]* They inserted a trach in his neck to help him breath. He was sent to Duke Hospital where the doctors kept him in ICU.
CW	*[Voice]* What about his parents?
HUMPHREY	*[Voice]* They kept fighting to take Val home. The doctors hired a personal nurse to teach them how to take care of him and use a feeding tube. He was born deaf and had no ears.

CW

[Voice] I am glad that he is alive. They are very blessed to have him, what will you do with him?

HUMPHREY

[Voice] I am going to help him learn.

CW

[Voice] Well, dear, please try to go back to sleep. Just plan what you will do for him. I am sure you will do your best.

HUMPHREY

[Voice] Thanks honey, I won't give up.

The next morning Humphrey arrives at Eagles Hall and finds Mrs. Cole at her desk.

COLE

[Voice] Good morning Humphrey, how are you doing?

HUMPHREY

[Voice] Good, but I didn't sleep well.

COLE

[Voice] What happened?

HUMPHREY

[Voice] I can't stop thinking about Val after reading the letter about his birth. It caused me to cry.

COLE

[Voice] I know how you feel. They told me the same thing when they visited my office. I am glad Mrs. Melvin sent the letter to you.

HUMPHREY

[Voice] Thanks. I have one question.

COLE

[Voice] Sure, ask me anything. What is it?

HUMPHREY

[Voice] Have you spanked Val? I am so sorry I asked you like that.

COLE

[Voice] It is okay, I know you care about Val. I often spanked him, but I decided not to spank him anymore after his mother told me about his birth.

HUMPHREY   *[Voice]* I understand. What will you do with
                    him when Val gets in trouble or behaves
                    badly?

COLE   *[Voice]* Well, I will call his parents if
                    something happens, and I will put Val in my
                    office to stay until he learns his lesson.

HUMPHREY   *[Voice]* I will do the same thing. Is it what
                    Mrs. Melvin wants us to do with him?

COLE   *[Voice]* That's right. I am glad you asked me
                    that question. You better go to your
                    classroom. Your students are waiting for
                    you.

HUMPHREY   *[Voice]* Okay, I need your help.

COLE   *[Voice]* Sure, what would you like me to do?

HUMPHREY   *[Voice]* Thanks, Cole. Tell me, how can I get
                    Val's trust?

COLE   *[Voice]* Just treat him nicely. You need to
                    make him do what you want him to do. If
                    the kids avoid him, you might pay attention
                    to him more. Please don't give up on him.

HUMPHREY   *[Voice]* I won't. Thanks for the advice.

COLE   *[Voice]* Welcome, anytime. Does Simmons
                    know about Val's birth? Do you have the
                    letter with you?

HUMPHREY   *[Voice]* I don't think she knows, but I will
                    give the letter to her and ask her to read it.

COLE   *[Voice]* That's a great idea. Good luck with
                    Val!

Humphrey walks in the hallway, when Simmons calls her name.

SIMMONS   *[Voice]* Humphrey, may I have a minute with you?

HUMPHREY   *[Voice]* Sure. Why don't we talk in your office?

SIMMONS   *[Voice]* Good idea, come on.

Simmons and Humphrey arrive at Simmons' office.

Simmons' office

HUMPHREY   *[Voice]* Okay. What do you want to talk about?

SIMMONS   *[Voice]* I hate to say this, but I'm thinking about moving Val to another classroom.

HUMPHREY   *[Voice]* Why?

SIMMONS   *[Voice]* Your students are still not getting along with him.

HUMPHREY   *[Voice]* I want to keep him in my class.

SIMMONS   *[Voice]* What about your students?

HUMPHREY   *[Voice]* I am going to work to make them be nice to him. I am going to help him learn.

SIMMONS   *[Voice]* How will you do that?

HUMPHREY   *[Voice]* I will get him to pay attention to me and listen to what I say. I will make him do everything for himself.

SIMMONS   *[Voice]* You want to do that for his parents and his brother?

HUMPHREY	*[Voice]* YES! I want to do it for myself too. Please give Val another chance to stay in my class.
SIMMONS	*[Voice]* I am still not sure if he trusts you, but I will allow him to stay in your class if he is better today. I will determine later today whether to move him to another classroom.
HUMPHREY	*[Voice]* He will trust me soon. You can check on us anytime you want.
SIMMONS	*[Voice]* Well, good luck. Go to your classroom.
HUMPHREY	*(Gives the letter to Simmons) [Voice]* Before I go, I want you to read the letter from Mrs. Melvin. I got it yesterday.
SIMMONS	*[Voice]* Really! What is it about?
HUMPHREY	*[Voice]* His birth. Go ahead, read it.

Humphrey leaves and Simmons holds the letter. She is about to throw it in the trash, but she changes her mind and reads it.

Humphrey teaches the kids how to write, but she is not pleased to see her students avoid Val, who sits alone.

Humphrey's classroom

HUMPHREY	*[Sign]* Kids, if you ignore him, I will pay attention to him more than to the rest of you.
STEPHEN	*[Sign]* Whatever, teach him if you want.
TRACI	*[Sign]* Why do you care about him? He is different from us.
HUMPHREY	*[Sign]* I care about him because he is special.

He was born with a birth defect. Why do you think Val is retarded?

MATTHEW

[Sign] The hole in his neck and his jaws. That's why.

The students laugh.

HUMPHREY

(Gets mad) [Sign] That's not funny! I want you to work on your language. I am going to teach Val now!

TRACI

[Sign] What will you teach him?

HUMPHREY

(Goes to Val's desk) [Sign] I will help him to write nicely. Get to work now. *(Turns to Val)* Val, I will teach you how to write.

VAL

[Sign] I am not good at writing; it is messy.

HUMPHREY

[Sign] Please let me help you write.

VAL

(Frowns at Humphrey) [Sign] Please don't touch me. Go away!

HUMPHREY

(Feels hurt) [Sign] It is time to practice your writing.

STEPHEN

[Sign] Nice try Humphrey! *(Laughs)*

HUMPHREY

(Points to the corner) [Sign] Go to the corner now! *(Stephen goes to the corner)*

Scene Five: Val Learns to Eat Pimento Cheese Sandwiches

In the lunchroom, the teachers and students are eating pimento cheese sandwiches for lunch, but Val doesn't eat his lunch and just drinks milk. Humphrey pulls the milk away and reminds Val to eat his lunch.

Eagles Hall lunchroom

HUMPHREY	*[Sign]* Val, why don't you eat your lunch?
VAL	*[Sign]* I don't want it.
HUMPHREY	*(Pulls milk away) [Sign]* Then no more milk for you.
VAL	*(Sounds upset) [Sign]* I want milk!
HUMPHREY	*(Points to Val's lunch) [Sign]* Eat your lunch now!
VAL	*(Gets mad) [Sign]* I won't.
HUMPHREY	*[Sign]* Too bad. You can't have it.
VAL	*(Cries) [Sign]* I am hungry!
HUMPHREY	*[Sign]* Then eat your sandwiches and soup.
VAL	*(Looks at his lunch) [Sign]* Are they good?
HUMPHREY	*[Sign]* Yes, they are. Please eat now.

Val holds his sandwich and looks at it.

HUMPHREY	*[Sign]* Are you going to eat this sandwich or not?
VAL	*[Sign]* Not sure.
HUMPHREY	*[Sign]* Well, let me try.
VAL	*[Sign]* You want the sandwich?

HUMPHREY   *(Grabs it and puts a piece into Val's mouth) [Sign]*
                           Like it?

*Val starts to get mad at Humphrey but he realizes the sandwich is very good.
He grabs it from Humphrey's hand and eats it.*

HUMPHREY   *[Sign]* Val, don't eat it too quickly!

VAL   *(Smiles at Humphrey) [Sign]* You are right. It is
                           good. I love it!

*Val eats another sandwich and looks at the soup. He eats it as Mrs.
Humphrey and the kids look on.*

STEPHEN   *[Sign]* Wow, he eats like a pig.

TRACI   *(Frowns at Stephen) [Sign]* Be quiet! Let Val
                           enjoy his lunch!

VAL   *(Gets up) [Sign]* Humphrey, they are good. I
                           want more sandwiches.

HUMPHREY   *[Sign]* Take it easy. Please sit down. I will get
                           more.

VAL   *[Sign]* I want more!

*Simmons shows up and asks Humphrey what's going on. Val eats more
pimento cheese sandwiches.*

SIMMONS   *[Voice]* Humphrey, what's going on with
                           Val?

HUMPHREY   *[Voice]* I made Val eat pimento cheese
                           sandwiches. He loves them. He asked for
                           more.

SIMMONS   *[Voice]* That's great. I was not sure if he
                           would trust you or not.

HUMPHREY   *[Voice]* Simmons, please give us some time.

He will trust me soon.

SIMMONS   *[Voice]* Alright. Good luck!

Humphrey's classroom

Humphrey decides to get Val to pay attention to her so she can teach him. The students are doing their work and don't understand why Humphrey pays attention to Val.

JUNIOR   *[Sign]* Humphrey, what are you doing with Val?

HUMPHREY   *[Sign]* I will teach him how to spell words for vegetables and fruits. Go back to work.

JUNIOR   *[Sign]* Okay, I hope we will keep him here.

HUMPHREY   *[Sign]* Thanks, Junior. *(Turns to Val)* Please finger spell the word.

VAL   *[Sign]* No!

HUMPHREY   *(Feels hurt) [Sigh]* Okay. I give up. I guess I am not going to teach you anymore because you won't listen to me.

VAL   *[Sign]* Why are you crying?

HUMPHREY   *[Sign]* You hurt my feelings! I am trying to help you to learn everything. If you don't want to learn, you have to move to another classroom.

VAL   *[Sign]* But I want to stay here.

HUMPHREY   *[Sign]* Then please let me teach you the lesson.

VAL   *[Sign]* Okay, teach me. I am so sorry.

HUMPHREY   *[Sign]* Thanks Val. Are you ready?

Val gets up and hugs Humphrey, then sits back in his chair. He smiles at her.

HUMPHREY   *[Sign]* What did you hug me for?

VAL   *[Sign]* Thanks for making me eat pimento cheese sandwiches. I love them.

HUMPHREY   *[Sign]* Aww. I am glad that you love them. Are you ready for a lesson?

VAL   *[Sign]* Yes.

HUMPHREY   *(Points to a card)* *[Sign]* What is it?

VAL   *[Sign]* T-o-m-a-t-o

HUMPHREY   *[Sign]* Good boy, what is this one?

VAL   *[Sign]* L-e-t-t-u-c-e

HUMPHREY   *[Sign]* Great. What about this one?

VAL   *[Sign]* B-e-a-n

HUMPHREY   *[Sign]* What about a long word?

VAL   *[Sign]* P-u-m-p-k-i-n

HUMPHREY   *[Sign]* Good boy. You did an amazing job!

VAL   *[Sign]* I want more!

HUMPHREY   *[Sign]* Sure. What about that?

VAL   *[Sign]* C-e-l-e-r-y

HUMPHREY   *[Sign]* Good job!

VAL   *[Sign]* Do they have sign names?

HUMPHREY	*[Sign]* I will tell you more tomorrow.
VAL	*[Sign]* I love spelling. It is fun!
HUMPHREY	*[Sign]* Kids, guess what?
TRACI	*[Sign]* What?
HUMPHREY	*[Sign]* Val knows how to spell the vegetables. He did an amazing job.

Humphrey runs to Simmons' office and tells her that Val finally listened to her. Humphrey invites Simmons to come to the classroom to see.

HUMPHREY	*[Voice]* Simmons, you have got to see Val. He learned something new. You will be surprised.
SIMMONS	*[Voice]* Please calm down. You sound too excited.
HUMPHREY	*[Sign]* I am so sorry. I just am excited!
SIMMONS	*[Voice]* Well, what did you teach him?
HUMPHREY	*[Sign]* Spelling. Come with me. You can watch us.

Humphrey fetches the flash cards and waves her hand at Val.

HUMPHREY	*[Sign]* Val, I want to show Simmons what I taught you.
VAL	*[Sign]* Okay. Teach me anything.
HUMPHREY	*[Sign]* Simmons, please look at us.
SIMMONS	*[Sign]* Alright, I am watching you.
HUMPHREY	*[Sign]* Are you ready Val?
VAL	*[Sign]* Yes.

HUMPHREY	*[Sign]* I have animal cards. Here is one. Spell the word.
VAL	*[Sign]* H-o-r-s-e *(Sign for a horse)*
HUMPHREY	*[Sign]* Good, here is another.
VAL	*[Sign]* C-o-w *(Sign for a cow)*
HUMPHREY	*[Sign]* Here is another.
VAL	*[Sign]* R-o-o-s-t-e-r *(Sign for a rooster)*
HUMPHREY	*[Voice]* What do you think? He finally did it!
SIMMONS	*(Smiles) [Voice to Humphrey and sign to Val]* That's wonderful. He did a great job. *(Turns to Val)* Do you want to stay in the classroom with Mrs. Humphrey?
VAL	*[Sign]* Yes. I want to stay here; I like Mrs. Humphrey.
SIMMONS	*[Voice]* Great to hear. It looks like he finally trusts you; he can stay in your classroom for the entire year.
HUMPHREY	*[Voice to Simmons and sign to Val]* Yay! I am very happy. *(Turns to Val)* Good news, you will stay here with me.
VAL	*[Sign]* I am very happy; I like it here.
HUMPHREY	*[Voice]* Me too. Thanks so much Simmons. It means everything to me.
SIMMONS	*[Voice]* Welcome, anytime. I need to tell you something important about his classmates.
HUMPHREY	*[Voice]* Sure, what about them?

SIMMONS	*[Voice]* Although you want to keep Val, you need to get his classmates to trust him and to accept him for who he is.
HUMPHREY	*[Voice]* I will try my best tomorrow.
SIMMONS	*[Voice]* It is time for Val to go to the dorm.
HUMPHREY	*[Sign]* Val, the class is dismissed. You may go to the dorm now. Have a good evening.
VAL	*(Hugs Humphrey) [Sign]* Goodbye Humphrey, I will see you tomorrow. *(He leaves)*
HUMPHREY	*(Smiles) [Voice]* He is very sweet. Isn't he?
SIMMONS	*[Voice]* Yes, he is. I am glad the two of you are finally getting along. Well, good luck getting your students to trust him.
HUMPHREY	*[Voice]* Sure, I will try my best. Thanks.

The next day Mrs. Humphrey teaches the kids a math problem but the kids still ignore Val. Mrs. Humphrey is upset to see them tell him to leave them alone. After lunch Traci goes to Humphrey's desk where she is correcting math problems.

TRACI	*(Walks to Humphrey's desk) [Sign]* Humphrey, what's wrong?
HUMPHREY	*[Sign]* I am disappointed that you all keep avoiding Val. None of you are nice to him. I want you all to accept him and be nice.
TRACI	*[Sign]* You are right. I have to be nice to him.
HUMPHREY	*[Sign]* Really, what changed your mind?
TRACI	*[Sign]* I saw his mother in the lobby. She is beautiful and sweet. I asked her who she was and she said she is Val's mother. Why is she

waiting in the lobby?

HUMPHREY	*[Sign]* She has to stay there until the class is finished.
TRACI	*[Sign]* Why don't we invite her to come here? They might be nice to Val after meeting his mother.
HUMPHREY	*[Sign]* Traci, you are right. I have to ask Simmons if Mrs. Melvin can stay here for a visit.
TRACI	*[Sign]* Okay.

Mrs. Humphrey turns on the intercom to talk to Miss Simmons.

HUMPHREY	*[Voice]* Hello Simmons, it is Humphrey. I have to ask you for permission.
SIMMONS	*[Voice]* Sure, what is it?
HUMPHREY	*[Voice]* Mrs. Melvin is in the lobby. I would like to know if you will allow her to come here for a visit.
SIMMONS	*[Voice]* But the class is not over, what do you need her for?
HUMPHREY	*[Voice]* I think meeting his mother will help the kids understand Val better. Traci met her in the lobby. She said his mother is beautiful and sweet.
SIMMONS	*[Voice]* That's a great idea. Although the kids are busy working, she might sit at your desk and watch everyone. Do you mind?
HUMPHREY	*[Voice]* It is fine with me and thanks so much!

SIMMONS   *[Voice]* Welcome. I will go to the lobby and tell her to go to your classroom.

HUMPHREY   *[Voice]* Why not let Val do that?

SIMMONS   *[Voice]* Good idea. Thanks for letting me know, talk to you later.

HUMPHREY   *[Sign]* Traci, you may tell Val that his mother is here and he can bring her here.

TRACI   *[Sign]* Sure, no problem. *(Turns to Val)* Your mother is in the lobby. You can bring her here to meet us.

VAL   *(Gets excited) [Sign]* Thanks, *(Turns to Humphrey)* is it okay if I get mama?

HUMPHREY   *[Sign]* Yes, you can go and get her.

VAL   *[Sign]* Thanks, I will be back. *(He leaves)*

STEPHEN   *(Raises his hand) [Sign]* Where did Val go?

HUMPHREY   *[Sign]* He is going to get his mother and bring her here. You will like her.

STEPHEN   *[Sign]* I bet his mother is ugly like him.

TRACI   *(Frowns) [Sign]* Stephen! Stop saying that! She is beautiful and sweet. I met her in the lobby.

CINDY   *[Sign]* Do we have to be nice to her?

TRACI   *[Sign]* Yes, she is Val's mother. Here they come.

VAL   *[Sign]* Hello. Here is my mother. She is here to meet you.

HUMPHREY   *[Sign]* Please tell her hello. Be nice.

THE KIDS   *[Sign]* Hello Val's mother.

BETTY   *[Sign to students and voice to Humphrey]* Hello. Nice to meet you. Val told me that you wanted me to stay here. Are you sure?

HUMPHREY   *[Voice]* Of course, you may sit at my desk. You can watch me teach them a math problem.

BETTY   *[Voice]* Thanks. Mrs. Humphrey, why doesn't Val introduce me to his classmates? Do you mind?

HUMPHREY   *[Voice to Betty and sign to Val]* Sure! *(Turns to Val)* Why don't you introduce your mother to your classmates?

VAL   *[Sign]* Okay, these are my classmates: Carolina, Traci, Cassandra, Corie, Junior, Kathy, Matthew, and Stephen. *(Points to each of his classmates)*

BETTY   *[Sign]* Thanks Val, have you made friends with them?

VAL   *[Sign]* Humphrey, do I have to tell her?

HUMPHREY   *[Sign]* Tell her yes; they are your friends.

VAL   *[Sign]* Yes, they are my friends. They are very nice.

STEPHEN   *[Sign]* Hey, he lied! We are not his friends!

HUMPHREY   *(Gets mad) [Sign]* Stephen, stop saying that! I don't want to upset his mother. Please be nice.

BETTY	*[Voice]* What did he say?
HUMPHREY	*[Voice]* Oh, Mrs. Melvin, he was just confused, but never mind.
BETTY	*[Sign]* Val, I am glad you made some friends.
CINDY	*[Sign]* Why did Val lie to his mother? His father is a pastor.
TRACI	*[Sign]* Take it easy. I don't want her to get upset if she finds out. We have to be nice to him and his mother.
KATHY	*[Sign]* Val, your mother is beautiful and sweet.
VAL	*[Sign]* Thanks so much, Kathy.
HUMPHREY	*[Sign to her students and voice to Betty]* Val, please sit down. Mrs. Melvin can watch me teach the math problem. *(Turns to Betty)* Mrs. Melvin, make yourself comfortable.
BETTY	*(Smiles) [Voice]* I am fine. Thanks, Mrs. Humphrey.

Humphrey teaches her students about addition and subtraction as Betty watches them.

On Monday morning, Mrs. Humphrey walks in the hallway, as Mrs. Cole interrupts her.

COLE	*[Voice]* Good morning Humphrey. Guess what?
HUMPHREY	*[Voice]* Good morning Cole. What is it?
COLE	*[Voice]* Val didn't cry or run away when his parents left. I know he trusts you. Have your students been nicer to him yet?

HUMPHREY   *[Voice]* Traci and Junior are two classmates who trust Val. I will work hard on the others.

COLE   *[Voice]* Great, I hope everything works out.

Eagles Hall Playground

Humphrey sees Val on the swing alone and goes to see her students who are playing ball together. She is disappointed they didn't invite Val to join them.

HUMPHREY   *[Sign]* Kids, why don't you let Val play ball with you?

STEPHEN   *[Sign]* If you want Val to play ball with us, it is fine with us.

HUMPHREY   *[Sign]* Please be nice to him. Where is he?

CAROLINA   *[Sign]* He is on the swing. I am going to get him.

HUMPHREY   *[Sign]* Okay. Go get him.

CAROLINA   *(Runs to the swing and tags Val) [Sign]* Val, would you like to play ball with us?

VAL   *[Sign]* Yes, I want to.

CAROLINA   *[Sign]* Come on and play with us.

Carolina and Val join the students playing ball. Humphrey forces them to let Val play. Val asks Stephen to throw the ball to him

Stephen in not pleased.

VAL   *[Sign]* Throw the ball to me.

STEPHEN   *[Sign]* No way. You are afraid of catching the ball.

VAL   *[Sign]* I will be okay.

JUNIOR   *[Sign]* Remember what Humphrey said.
                    Throw the ball to him, and be nice to him.

CINDY   *[Sign]* He is playing with us so throw the ball
                    to him.

STEPHEN   *(Gets mad) [Sign]* Okay, I am going to throw
                    the ball to Val now!

*Stephen throws the ball hard to Val, but the ball hits his front tooth and
starts to bleed.*

TRACI   *[Sign]* Stephen! You hit his tooth.

CINDY   *[Sign]* I am going to get Humphrey.

JUNIOR   *(Pushes Stephen hard) [Sign]* I don't like the way
                    you treat Val. *(Turns to Val)* Are you okay?

VAL   *[Sign]* My tooth is bleeding; I need to go to
                    the infirmary.

JUNIOR   *[Sign]* Take it easy, here comes Humphrey.

HUMPHREY   *[Runs and hugs Val]* Oh Val! Your tooth is
                    bleeding, who did this?

JUNIOR   *[Sign]* Stephen did it.

HUMPHREY   *[Sign]* I want you to go to Simmons' office
                    now! *(Grabs Stephen's arm)* Val, come on.

VAL   *[Sign]* I need to go to the infirmary.

HUMPHREY   *[Sign]* Okay, we will go there. Kids, go to the
                    classroom. I will get someone to watch you.

STEPHEN   *[Sign]* Am I being punished?

HUMPHREY	*[Sign]* Yes, you threw the ball at him hard. You have to go to Simmons' office to be disciplined.

Humphrey drops Stephen by Simmons' office and brings Val to the infirmary. The nurse checks on his tooth to make sure it is okay.

Infirmary

HUMPHREY	*[Voice]* Barnes, did Val's tooth fall out?
JEAN	*[Voice]* Almost. It is numb. He is holding a cloth on his tooth until it stops bleeding.
HUMPHREY	*[Voice]* Thanks. I am glad that he is alright.
JEAN	*[Voice to Humphrey and sign to Val]* Here Val comes. Val, be careful. Don't let anyone throw the ball hard again.
VAL	*[Sign]* Okay.
HUMPHREY	*[Sign]* Come on, let's go back to the classroom.
VAL	*[Sign]* Are you going to tell mama and papa what happened to my tooth?
HUMPHREY	*[Sign]* Yes, I have to tell them. They need to know.
VAL	*[Sign]* Okay. What about Stephen? Will you tell them that he did it to me?
HUMPHREY	*[Sign]* I don't think so. I don't want to upset them. I will just tell them your tooth got hit. That's all. Please don't tell them what Stephen did to you.
VAL	*[Sign]* Okay, I won't.

HUMPHREY   *[Sign]* Good boy, please hold the cloth to your tooth.

Humphrey's Classroom

After class, while Mrs. Humphrey clears the class table, Mrs. Dawson shows up.

DAWSON   *[Voice]* Hey Humphrey, can I come in?

HUMPHREY   *[Voice]* Hey Beth, you can come in. How is your class doing?

DAWSON   *[Voice]* Doing great, how about your class?

HUMPHREY   *[Voice]* Doing okay, but I had a rough day today.

DAWSON   *[Voice]* Really? Something happen with Val?

HUMPHREY   *[Voice]* Yes, his tooth got hit. Stephen threw the ball hard at him; it was bleeding. He is okay now.

DAWSON   *[Voice]* I am so sorry. Did you get your students to accept him yet?

HUMPHREY   *[Voice]* Junior and Traci are two. Junior found out Val's father is a pastor and Traci met Val's mother in the lobby. They were nice to him after that.

DAWSON   *[Voice]* That's nice. Do you think you will get the others to like him?

HUMPHREY   *[Voice]* I am working on that.

DAWSON   *[Voice]* You okay? You look very worried.

HUMPHREY   *[Voice]* Yes, I am worried about him. I don't want him to get hurt.

DAWSON   *[Voice]* I think you need to go home and
                relax. If you are still worried about Val, why
                don't you check on him before going home?

HUMPHREY   *[Voice]* I am planning on it, thanks.

Humphrey goes to the office and finds Simmons getting ready to go home.

HUMPHREY   *[Voice]* Hey Simmons, is it okay if I check on
                Val before going home?

SIMMONS   *[Voice]* Sure you can. You care about Val?

HUMPHREY   *[Voice]* Yes, he is very special to me. Have a
                good evening.

SIMMONS   *[Voice]* Okay, you too.

Scene Six: Val Meets Humphrey's Husband and Sons

*Humphrey goes to the dorm and finds Val and his group at the playground.
She looks at them through the window and sees Val sitting against the wall.
Humphrey becomes upset and goes to Cole's office.*

Cole's Office

HUMPHREY   *[Voice]* Hello Mrs. Cole, I need to tell you
                something.

COLE   *[Voice]* Sure, what is it?

HUMPHREY   *[Voice]* I saw the kids playing outside, but
                Val was sitting alone. Is something wrong
                with him? Is he being punished?

COLE   *[Voice]* No, they just don't want to play with
                him.

HUMPHREY   *[Voice]* I know, I would like to invite him for
                dinner with me and my family. It will make

him very happy. I will bring him back
tonight.

COLE   *[Voice]* That's sweet of you, but you have to
                      ask his parents for permission.

HUMPHREY   *[Voice]* Okay, I will call them now, but I
                      need their number.

COLE   *(Shows the phone number)* *[Voice]* Here is the
                      number. You can use my phone to call Mrs.
                      Melvin.

HUMPHREY   *[Voice]* Thanks Cole. *(Dials the number)*

BETTY   *[Voice]* Hello this is the Melvin residence.
                      Who is this?

HUMPHREY   *[Voice]* Hello Mrs. Melvin, it is me, Mary Sue
                      Humphrey. I would like to ask you if I can
                      take your son to my place for dinner with
                      me and my family this evening. I will bring
                      him back tonight.

BETTY   *[Voice]* Oh Mrs. Humphrey, how sweet of
                      you! How is Val doing?

HUMPHREY   *[Voice]* He is doing fine. He has begun to
                      accept me and lets me teach him things. He
                      keeps hugging me after class every day.

BETTY   *[Voice]* That is great to hear! He knows you
                      care about him.

HUMPHREY   *[Voice]* Yes, I realize that. Is it okay with you
                      and your husband if I take him to my place
                      for dinner?

BETTY   *[Voice]* He is at work now, but I am sure it is
                      fine. What are you having for supper?

HUMPHREY	*[Voice]* Spaghetti and meat sauce.
BETTY	*[Voice]* That is Val's favorite food! Please cut it into small bites before he eats. It is very nice of you to invite him. Tell Cole you are allowed to take him. I hope you and your family enjoy having him for dinner. Please send my love to him. Thanks so much; you are sweet and kind.
HUMPHREY	*[Voice]* Great! Thanks so much for the compliment. I will cut his food and take care of him. Have a good evening, bye.
COLE	*[Voice]* Approved?
HUMPHREY	*[Voice]* Yes. I am going to get Val now. Thanks so much.
COLE	*[Voice]* I hope you enjoy your evening with him. I have to go with you because I need to let Miss Bass know you will take him to your place for dinner.

Eagles Hall Playground

Cole and Humphrey go to the playground. Cole tells Miss Bass to let Humphrey take Val. They go to her car as the boys watch them.

JUNIOR	*[Sign]* Where is Val? I don't see him here.
STEPHEN	*[Sign]* Who cares?
JUNIOR	*[Sign]* You don't like him?
STEPHEN	*[Sign]* So what. He is ugly.
MATTHEW	*[Sign]* I saw Humphrey take Val somewhere.
STEPHEN	*[Sign]* Yes!

MATTHEW	*[Sign]* Why are you happy?
STEPHEN	*[Sign]* Yes, we got of rid of him, so we won't see him again.
JUNIOR	*[Sign]* I don't think so.
STEPHEN	*[Sign]* What?
JUNIOR	*[Sign]* I think she is taking him to her place for dinner because she feels bad for him.
MATTHEW	*[Sign]* I think Val is her favorite student. She is very nice to him.
STEPHEN	*[Sign]* You two shut up! We will find out soon.

The Humphrey Residence

Humphrey takes Val to her house and they go inside. Val looks around as Humphrey checks her mail.

HUMPHREY	*[Sign]* Val, welcome to the Humphrey residence, make yourself comfortable while I fix supper for everyone.
VAL	*[Sign]* Thanks, why did you bring me here?
HUMPHREY	*[Sign]* I wanted to invite you to eat supper with me and my family. I want you to have a great time with us.
VAL	*[Sign]* I am happy now. Where are your husband and your sons?
HUMPHREY	*[Sign]* They will be here soon. Please be patient.
VAL	*[Sign]* Okay. What are we having for supper?

HUMPHREY	*[Sign]* Spaghetti and meat sauce!
VAL	*(Jumps excitedly)* *[Sign]* That is my favorite!
HUMPHREY	*[Sign]* I know you are excited. Please take it easy.
VAL	*(Hugs Humphrey)* *[Sign]* Yes! I am very excited. Thanks so much. You are the best!
HUMPHREY	*[Sign]* Aww. You can watch TV if you want; I have to fix supper before they arrive.
VAL	*[Sign]* Okay. I want to watch The Brady Bunch.
HUMPHREY	*(Changes the channel)* *[Sign]* Here it is. Enjoy the show, talk to you later.
VAL	*[Sign]* Okay thanks!

CW arrives at the Humphrey residence and is surprised to see Val there.

| CW | *[Voice]* Hello honey, I am home. *(Looks at Val)* Is he one of your students? |
| HUMPHREY | *[Voice]* Hello CW! Yes, this is my student. His name is Val Melvin. He is here to have supper with us. |

Val gets up and waves at Mr. Humphrey

HUMPHREY	*[Sign]* This is my husband, CW Humphrey.
VAL	*[Sign]* Hi Mr. Humphrey, nice to meet you. She invited me here for supper.
HUMPHREY	*[Voice]* He is a sweet and kind boy isn't he?
CW	*[Voice]* Yes, he is. Mary Sue, let's go to our room, I need you to explain why Val is here.

HUMPHREY	*[Voice to CW and sign to Val]* Okay, CW. *(Turns to Val)* We need to talk in private. I will be back. Enjoy the show.
CW	*[Voice]* Mary Sue, why did you invite him here without my permission? You should have asked me first.
HUMPHREY	*[Voice]* I am very sorry. I feel awful for him because the kids keep avoiding him. I can't help it. If you want me to take him back, I will.
CW	*[Voice]* Wait a minute. I saw he has a hole in his neck. Was it him that his mother wrote a letter about?
HUMPHREY	*[Voice]* Right, it is him.
CW	*[Voice]* Oh I got it. Did you ask his parents for permission to bring him here?
HUMPHREY	*[Voice]* Yes. They said it was fine.
CW	*[Voice]* Okay, I would like to talk to him.
HUMPHREY	*[Sign]* Val, my husband wants to talk to you now.
VAL	*[Sign]* Okay.
CW	*[Voice]* Tell him he is welcome to have supper with us.
HUMPHREY	*[Voice]* You want me to tell him to stay with us for supper?
CW	*[Voice]* Of course. I read the letter. I feel the same way you do. Val can stay here.
HUMPHREY	*[Sign]* Val, my husband said you are welcome

to stay here for dinner.

VAL

(Smiles and hugs him) *[Sign]* Thanks so much, Mr. Humphrey

HUMPHREY

[Voice] I am so sorry. He loves hugging people when he greets them.

CW

[Voice] It is okay. He is sweet.

THOMAS

[Voice] Mom, we are home. We are sorry we are late.

BLAINE

[Voice] Look at the boy! Who is this?

THOMAS

[Voice] Mommy, why don't you introduce us to the boy? Is it one of your students?

HUMPHREY

[Voice] Hello boys, this is Val Melvin. He is here to have supper with us.

BLAINE

[Voice] That's nice. Why don't you introduce him to us?

HUMPHREY

[Sign] Val, I would like you to meet my sons.

Val waves at Thomas and Blaine.

HUMPHREY

[Sign] This is Thomas. He is older.

VAL

[Sign] Hello Thomas.

HUMPHREY

[Sign] This is Blaine he is younger.

VAL

[Sign] Hello Blaine. You remind me of my brother.

BLAINE

[Voice] His brother?

HUMPHREY

[Voice and sign] Yes, he has an older brother named Alan. Please keep him company

while I finish cooking supper.

VAL   *[Sign]* Can they sign like you?

HUMPHREY   *[Sign]* A little; they are just learning sign language.

THOMAS   *[Voice]* Ask Val if he would like to walk with us around the neighborhood.

HUMPHREY   *[Sign]* Val, they want you to walk with them around the neighborhood.

VAL   *[Sign]* That's sweet. Okay, I will go with you.

HUMPHREY   *[Sign and voice]* Have fun. Please be careful, and don't let him get lost.

BLAINE   *[Voice]* Okay. We will keep eye on him.

Humphrey goes back to preparing dinner and after a while calls her husband and sons for supper.

HUMPHREY   *[Voice and sign]* It is time for supper now.

VAL   *[Sign]* Humphrey, may I go to the bathroom and wash my hands?

HUMPHREY   *[Sign]* Good idea. Do that.

HUMPHREY   *[Sign]* You can sit next to me if you want

VAL   *[Sign]* Sure, thanks. The food looks good to me.

HUMPHREY   *[Voice]* Oh no, I almost forgot something.

CW   *[Voice]* What is it?

HUMPHREY   *[Voice]* Val's mother told me to cut his food before he eats. Excuse me.

| VAL | *[Sign]* Where is the cheese? I need it. |
| THOMAS | *[Voice]* Got it. Here it is. |

Val eats spaghetti and meat sauce quickly and Mrs. Humphrey tells him to eat slowly. Val looks happy as he eats his supper. Soon his plate is empty.

| HUMPHREY | *[Sign]* How did you like it? |
| VAL | *(Thumbs up) [Sign]* It was very good; thanks so much! |

After dinner Val goes to Thomas and Blaine's room while they do homework. Humphrey shows up and stops him.

HUMPHREY	*[Sign]* No Val, please don't bother them. They are doing homework.
THOMAS	*[Voice]* It is okay. Let him look around here. I like him.
BLAINE	*[Voice]* The room might remind him of Alan.
HUMPHREY	*[Voice]* He can, for a short time, then I will take him back to school.
VAL	*(Points to a poster) [Sign]* Alan has one like that.
BLAINE	*[Voice]* Awesome, he must be a KISS fan too.
HUMPHREY	*[Sign]* Val, it is time to take you back to school. Come on.

Val doesn't move. He thinks about Alan.

| THOMAS | *[Voice]* What is wrong with him? |
| HUMPHREY | *[Sign]* Come on Val. |

VAL   *(Points to Blaine) [Sign]* Blaine, *(Points to Thomas)* Thomas.

HUMPHREY   *[Sign]* Right! You can say goodbye to them before we leave.

Val puts an "A" on his forehead as they watch.

BLAINE   *[Voice]* Mommy, what is he signing?

HUMPHREY   *[Sign]* Val, what is that sign?

VAL   *(Finger spells) [Sign]* A-L-A-N

HUMPHREY   *[Sign]* Do you have a sign name for him?

VAL   *(Tears) [Sign]* Yes, I have a sign name for him.

THOMAS   *[Voice]* He must miss his brother.

HUMPHREY   *[Voice to her sons and sign to Val]* That's right. He will see his brother this weekend. Val, it is time to go back to school. Say goodbye to Thomas and Blaine.

VAL   *(Hugs Thomas and Blaine) [Sign]* Goodbye Thomas and Blaine

BLAINE   *[Voice]* Aww sweet. He is very nice. Hope to see you again.

THOMAS   *[Voice]* Please visit us again.

HUMPHREY   *[Sign]* Val, come with me.

VAL   *[Sign]* Your husband and your sons are very nice. I would like to see them again.

HUMPHREY   *[Sign]* Thanks, you will see them again.

Humphrey takes Val to Eagles Hall. They see Cole at her desk. Val dances

happily and Cole realizes he had a great time.

COLE   *[Sign]* Hey Val, did you have a good time
                with Mrs. Humphrey and her family?

VAL   *[Sign]* Yes. I ate spaghetti and meat sauce. It
                was very good. Her family is nice and sweet.

COLE   *[Sign]* Great to hear. I am glad you had a
                good time. Thanks Humphrey, for taking
                Val. We need to go to the infirmary for your
                trach to be cleaned.

VAL   *[Sign]* Finished.

HUMPHREY   *[Voice]* I took him there before bringing him
                here.

COLE   *[Voice to Humphrey and sign to Val]* Oh, thanks
                so much. Val, it is time to go to the dorm
                and get a bath. What do you say to Mrs.
                Humphrey?

VAL   *(Turns to Humphrey and hugs her) [Sign]* Thanks
                so much for dinner! I had a great time.
                Good night and see you tomorrow. *(Goes to
                the dorm)*

COLE   *[Voice]* He is a very sweet boy, isn't he?

HUMPHREY   *[Voice]* Yes, he is very sweet. You were right
                about him.

COLE   *[Voice]* What do you mean?

HUMPHREY   *[Voice]* You told me not to give up on him
                until I helped him learn.

COLE   *[Voice]* Right! It is great to hear you won his
                trust. It is the first step.

HUMPHREY	*[Voice]* Yeah. I will teach him more lessons. Good night

The next morning Val and his classmates arrive at the classroom. Humphrey asks them to take a seat. Val goes to Mrs. Humphrey and hugs her as the students look at them.

HUMPHREY	*[Sign]* Thanks, Val please sit down.
TRACI	*[Sign]* What did Val hug you for? He must like you.
STEPHEN	*[Sign]* Traci, I know why. Val is very happy because she took him to her house for supper with her and her family.
TRACI	*[Sign]* Oh, Humphrey. You didn't invite us to join you for supper. It is unfair!
CINDY	*[Sign]* I agree. Shame on you!
HUMPHREY	*[Sign]* Take it easy, let me explain everything.
SIMMONS	*(Shows up) [Voice]* Good morning Humphrey.
HUMPHREY	*[Voice]* Good morning Simmons, what's going on?
SIMMONS	*(Looks at Val) [Voice]* How is Val doing? He looks very happy.
HUMPHREY	*(Smiles nervously) [Voice]* Yes, he is doing great.
STEPHEN	*(Tags Simmons) [Sign]* Simmons, I have to tell you why Val is happy.
SIMMONS	*[Sign]* Really, what is it?
STEPHEN	*[Sign]* She took him to her house for supper with her and her family. She didn't invite us

to join them.

SIMMONS	*(Turns to Humphrey)* *[Voice]* Humphrey, is this true?
HUMPHREY	*[Voice]* Yes, let me explain everything.
SIMMONS	*(Gets mad)* *[Voice]* Go to my office now.
HUMPHREY	*[Voice]* What about the kids?
SIMMONS	*(Calls Dawson)* *[Voice]* Mrs. Dawson, please watch the kids while Humphrey is in my office.
HUMPHREY	*[Sign]* Kids, please behave yourself for Mrs. Dawson.
SIMMONS	*[Sign]* Val, I want you come to my office with us too.
HUMPHREY	*[Voice]* Simmons, Val did nothing wrong. I just invited him to come to my place.
SIMMONS	*[Voice to Humphrey and sign to Val]* I know but you didn't invite the other kids, *(Grabs Val's arm)* come with me. *(They leave to go to her office as Stephen laughs)*
TRACI	*[Sign]* Stephen, you got Humphrey and Val in trouble. Shame on you. It is not nice.
STEPHEN	*[Sign]* You like Val?
TRACI	*[Sign]* Yes, why?
STEPHEN	*[Sign]* Well, I am going to tell everyone how much you like him. They will make fun of you.
JUNIOR	*[Sign]* Stop teasing Traci! I am with her.

STEPHEN   *[Sign]* I can't believe you two are on the ugly
                      duckling's side.

JUNIOR   *[Sign]* Shut up Stephen. I have to be nice to
                      him because he is a pastor's son.

TRACI   *[Sign]* His mommy brought cupcakes to us.
                      She is sweet and beautiful.

STEPHEN   *[Sign]* Well, are you two his friends or not?

Traci and Junior look at each other and turn to Stephen.

TRACI   *[Sign]* Yes, we are his friends.

STEPHEN   *[Sign]* Ask the others if they are Val's friends.

*The other classmates look at each other and agree with Stephen. They say they
are not Val's friend. Junior and Traci are heartbroken.*

JUNIOR   *[Sign]* None of them are his friends. What
                      are we doing?

TRACI   *[Sign]* Wait and see.

*Humphrey and Val arrive at the Principal's office. Val is scared of
Simmons.*

Simmons' Office

VAL   *[Sign]* Please hold me. I am scared of
                      Simmons.

HUMPHREY   *[Sign]* Take it easy, I am here with you.
                      Please sit down while I talk to Simmons.

VAL   *[Sign]* I want to be with you. I feel safe with
                      you.

SIMMONS   *[Voice]* That's it. I will spank him and teach
                      him a lesson.

HUMPHREY	*[Voice]* Don't do that. I invited him because nobody is friends with Val, so I took him to my house.
SIMMMONS	*[Voice]* Wait a minute. You checked on how he was doing before you left for home?
HUMPHREY	*[Voice]* Yes. I wanted to check on him. I care about him.
SIMMONS	*[Voice]* Well, his houseparent would take care of him. He is your student, not your son. Did Mrs. Cole know about this?
HUMPHREY	*[Voice]* Yes, I called his parents for permission. They said it was okay for me to take him. Look at him, he had a great time with me and my family.
SIMMONS	*[Sign]* Okay, Val, did your parents know Humphrey took you to her house for supper?

The phone rings but Simmons ignores it and keeps asking Val if his parents knew or not. Val doesn't say anything.

HUMPHREY	*(Points to the phone) [Voice]* Simmons, why don't you answer the phone?
SIMMONS	*(Gets mad at Humphrey) [Voice]* I know! I need an answer from Val, now!

The phone still rings.

HUMPHREY	*[Voice]* What if it is an important call?
SIMMONS	*(Still upset) [Voice]* Okay! Okay! I am going to get it! *(Answers the phone)* Hello, this is Principal Simmons' office. Who is this?

It is a call from Val's mother and she tells Simmons that Humphrey called

*her for permission yesterday. Mrs. Melvin asks her if it is alright with
Simmons. Simmons clears her throat.*

SIMMONS   *(Sighs) [Voice]* Okay, Mrs. Melvin. Thanks so
                 much for letting me know. See you then.
                 Bye. *(She hangs up and turns to Humphrey)* I
                 think I better let you two go. I am so sorry.

HUMPHREY   *(Smiles) [Voice]* Thanks so much. I am glad
                 that she called you.

VAL   *[Sign]* Who was on the phone?

SIMMONS   *[Sign]* It was your mother. She said Mrs.
                 Humphrey called her for permission. I am so
                 sorry. You are free to go now.

HUMPHREY   *[Voice to Simmons and sign to Val]* Thanks so
                 much Simmons. *(Turns to Val)* Val, come
                 with me.

*Mrs. Humphrey and Val walk in the class hallway. Val notices that his
teacher holds his hand.*

HUMPHREY   *[Sign]* I am glad your mother called Miss
                 Simmons.

VAL   *[Sign]* Me too. *(Looks at their hands held)* You
                 are holding my hand.

HUMPHREY   *(Laughs) [Sign]* You know how much I care
                 about you.

Val looks at his teacher and smiles.

Scene Seven: "I Don't Want to Lose Val!"

Humphrey and the students are at the table eating in the lunchroom. Humphrey is mad at her students for what they did to her and Val. They are having greens, corn, and sausage.

The Eagles Hall Lunchroom

TRACI	*[Sign]* Humphrey, you okay?
HUMPHREY	*[Sign]* I am doing fine. Go eat your lunch.
TRACI	*[Sign]* You look upset. You are mad with Stephen.
HUMPHREY	*[Sign]* What are you talking about?
TRACI	*[Sign]* Stephen got you two into trouble. Is everything alright?
STEPHEN	*[Sign]* Traci! Stop talking behind my back!
HUMPHREY	*[Sign]* Stephen go eat your lunch. *(Turns to Traci)* I don't want to talk about that. Please eat your lunch now.
TRACI	*[Sign]* Okay, I am sorry.
VAL	*(Touches Humphrey) [Sign]* Humphrey.
HUMPHREY	*[Sign]* Yes?
VAL	*[Sign]* I am not sure if I can eat the sausage.
HUMPHREY	*[Sign]* Eat it. It is very good for you.
VAL	*[Sign]* Do you want me to eat it?
HUMPHREY	*[Sign]* Yes, go eat your lunch.

Val looks at the sausage and eats it, but he is unable to swallow it.

JUNIOR   *[Sign]* Humphrey, something is wrong with
                  him, he is acting strange.

HUMPHREY   *[Sign]* Val, you okay?

Val doesn't move and points to his neck.

HUMPHREY   *[Sign]* Did you swallow the food yet?

Val still points to his neck and faints.

HUMPHREY   *(Screams) [Sign]* Oh no Val! Let me help you!

Humphrey holds Val and tries to get the food out of his mouth but Val feels dizzy. The classmates look at him and worry.

SIMMONS   *(Runs to the table) [Voice]* Humphrey, what
                  happened to Val?

HUMPHREY   *[Voice]* We need to get him to the infirmary.
                  He ate sausage, but he couldn't swallow it. It
                  is stuck in his throat, we need help!

SIMMONS   *[Voice]* Oh no! We need two men to take
                  him. Farmer, Massey, can you pick him up
                  and get him to the infirmary?

Massey and Farmer pick Val up and take him to the infirmary as everyone looks on.

HUMPHREY   *[Voice]* Please let me go with them. I want to
                  be with Val, he needs me now.

SIMMONS   *[Voice]* But you have to stay with the kids.
                  The nurses will take care of everything.

HUMPHREY   *[Voice]* Aw, please!

TRACI   *(Tags Simmons) [Sign]* Please let Humphrey go
                  with them. She cares about him. You can
                  stay with us.

SIMMONS	*[Sign to Traci voice to Simmons]* I understand. *(Turns to Humphrey)* Okay, go with them. Please let me know how he is doing.
HUMPHREY	*[Sign and voice]* Okay, I will. Thanks so much. *(She leaves)*
STEPHEN	*[Sign]* Wow. Is he going to die?
JUNIOR	*(Punches Stephen's shoulder) [Sign]* Stop saying that! We need to pray for him to be alright.
STEPHEN	*[Sign]* Simmons! Junior hit my shoulder!
SIMMONS	*[Sign]* You better stop that!
JUNIOR	*[Sign]* I am so sorry. I didn't mean it.

Mrs. Humphrey rushes to the infirmary and goes to the doctor's office. The nurses are having a hard time getting the sausage out of Val's mouth as Humphrey looks on.

JEAN	*[Voice]* Humphrey, please go away. We have a lot to do.
HUMPHREY	*[Voice]* But I was with him when it happened. I am worried about him; he needs me now.
FARMER	*[Voice]* Please let her stay with us. Val kept asking about her. We need to do something to get the food out.
MASSEY	*[Voice]* Try drinking water.
JEAN	*[Sign]* Val, please drink water.
VAL	*(Drinks the water) [Sign]* I feel dizzy.
FARMER	*[Voice]* This is not working! What are we going to do?

JEAN	*[Voice]* I must think of something. I need to get Q-tips.
FARMER	*[Voice]* I don't think so. Think of something else.
MASSEY	*[Voice]* Come on, we need to keep Val alive.
HUMPHREY	*(Looks at the suction machine) [Voice]* Why don't you use this?

Carol Farmer and Jean Barnes look at each other and agree with Humphrey.

JEAN	*[Voice]* Massey, take Val to the sink. I will feed his tube down his throat while you hold him.
MASSEY	*[Voice]* Sure, go on.
HUMPHREY	*[Sign]* Val, please breathe when Jean inserts your trach.

Val chokes and the food comes out.

FARMER	*[Voice]* Wow. It worked out. Thank the Lord!
HUMPHREY	*(Pats Val's back and hugs him) [Sign]* You did an amazing job, Val. I was very scared.
VAL	*[Sign]* I need a drink.
HUMPHREY	*[Sign]* Jean, he needs water to drink.
JEAN	*(Gives Val a drink) [Sign]* Here it is, drink it. Good boy.

Val drinks water as everyone looks at him.

MASSEY	*[Sign]* I am glad it is over. Val, I am glad you are alright.

VAL	[Sign] Thanks. (He faints)
MASSEY	(Looks surprised) [Voice] Is Val alright?
JEAN	[Voice] Yes, he needs rest for now. Let me put Val to bed.
HUMPHREY	[Voice] Let me help you please.

Jean and Humphrey take him to the infirmary bed. Val falls asleep as Humphrey puts the blanket on him.

JEAN	[Voice] Thanks for your help. I am glad you were here with us. I think you better go to Eagles Hall.
HUMPHREY	[Voice] I can't leave him like this. Do you mind if I stay here for a while?
JEAN	[Voice] What about your other students?
HUMPHREY	[Voice] Don't worry, someone is watching them. Please let me stay with him for a while.
JEAN	[Voice] I understand how you feel. You can stay here with him if you want.
HUMPHREY	[Voice] Thanks so much. I appreciate that.

Humphrey sits on the chair next to Val who is lying on the bed. She falls asleep. Later Simmons comes to the infirmary and looks at Humphrey and Val. Simmons touches Humphrey to wake her up.

SIMMONS	[Voice] Wake up Humphrey.
HUMPHREY	[Voice] Oh, hello Simmons. I am so sorry I was with Val for a while. I was very worried.
SIMMONS	[Voice] It's okay, he's sleeping. How did they get the sausage out?

HUMPHREY	*[Voice]* They used the suction machine to make him cough and it came out.
SIMMONS	*[Voice]* I was very scared for him, but I am glad he is alright. I need to call his parents and let them know what happened. I don't know what to say. They may be upset.
HUMPHREY	*[Voice]* You don't have to call them. Wait until Mrs. Melvin arrives on Friday.
SIMMONS	*[Voice]* You are right. I need to call her to bring her and her husband in for a meeting.
HUMPHREY	*[Voice]* About what happened today?
SIMMONS	*[Voice]* That's right, I hope everything is going to be alright. It is time for you go back to the classroom.
HUMPHREY	*[Voice]* I can't leave him like this.
SIMMONS	*[Voice]* I know, but Val is resting. The nurse will take care of him. Your students need you now, they kept asking about Val.
HUMPHREY	*[Voice]* Really, what did they say?
SIMMONS	*[Voice]* They cried and were very worried about him. I think you need to talk to them.
HUMPHREY	*[Voice]* Okay. I will go. *(Pats Val's head)* Val, I love you.
SIMMONS	*[Voice]* That's sweet, but he can't hear what you say.
HUMPHREY	*[Voice]* I know, but he will realize how much I love him.
SIMMONS	*[Voice]* I understand, let's go.

HUMPHREY	*[Voice]* Simmons?
SIMMONS	*[Voice]* Yes?
HUMPHREY	*[Voice]* Can I check on him after school? Please?
SIMMONS	*[Voice]* Sure, you can.
HUMPHREY	*[Voice]* Thanks so much Simmons.

Simmons comforts Humphrey as they leave the infirmary and go to Eagles Hall.

In Humphrey's classroom the students are very worried about Val and feel bad about treating him badly. They are anxious for Humphrey's return.

Humphrey's Classroom

CAROLINA	*[Sign]* Traci, I am so sorry. You are right.
TRACI	*[Sign]* About Val?
CAROLINA	*[Sign]* Yes, we have to be nice. We will tell him how we are sorry we were mean to him.
TRACI	*[Sign]* Will you be his friend?
CAROLINA	*[Sign]* Not sure.
TRACI	*[Sign]* Not sure? You were very scared about what happened to him.
CAROLINA	*[Sign]* I know I don't want him to die.
TRACI	*[Sign]* It looks like you care about him.
CAROLINA	*[Sign]* Right, I will be his friend. What about the others?
TRACI	*[Sign]* Cindy? Do you want to be his friend?

CINDY	*[Sign]* Yes.
TRACI	*[Sign]* What about you, Cassandra?
CASSANDRA	*[Sign]* I don't know what to say. I don't talk to him much. He tried to hug me, but I was not comfortable hugging.
TRACI	*[Sign]* He can't help it. He loves hugging anyone who cares about him. Do you care about him?
CASSANDRA	*[Sign]* Is he all right?
TRACI	*[Sign]* Wait until Humphrey arrives.
KATHY	*[Sign]* Traci, I accept, I am his friend.
TRACI	*[Sign]* Look, Kathy wants to be Val's friend.
CASSANDRA	*[Sign]* I have to be nice to him, then we can be friends.
TRACI	*[Sign]* Good, what about you Corie?
CORIE	*[Sign]* Well, I like him, but he acts strange. I guess I will give him a chance.
TRACI	*[Sign]* Thanks so much Corie. *(Turns to Junior)* Junior, you need to help Matthew and Stephen be Val's friends. They don't listen to me.
JUNIOR	*[Sign]* Don't worry, I will take care of them. *(Turns to Matthew and Stephen)* I want you to be Val's friend.
MATTHEW	*[Sign]* Aww. Why would I be his friend?
STEPHEN	*[Sign]* Wait and see, we have to check on him.

JUNIOR	[Sign] I guess I need to ask Humphrey to tell us everything about Val. I believe that will change their minds.
TRACI	[Sign] Okay. Here Humphrey comes.

Humphrey comes in and walks slowly as the classmates look at her.

HUMPHREY	[Sign] Hello students. I just came back from the infirmary. I am very tired.
JUNIOR	[Sign] Why don't you sit down and relax?
TRACI	[Sign] Here is a glass of water, please drink.
HUMPHREY	(Sits down and drinks water) [Sign] Thanks so much. I appreciate your concern.
CINDY	[Sign] How is Val doing? Is he alright?
HUMPHREY	[Sign] He is okay now. The sausage came out of his throat. He is better and is sleeping.
CAROLINA	[Sign] I am glad that he is better. Why don't we go to the infirmary to see how he is?
HUMPHREY	[Sign] That's very sweet of you, but not now. He is resting. He had a hard time today. It is my fault.
TRACI	[Sign] Your fault?
HUMPHREY	[Sign] His mother kept telling me to cut his food for him before he eats. I forgot today.
TRACI	[Sign] Please don't feel bad. We will help you.
HUMPHREY	[Sign] Help me?
TRACI	[Sign] Yes, we are going to help you to teach

him. That's why you pay attention to him.

CINDY   *[Sign]* We can be his friends and make him very happy.

HUMPHREY   *[Sign]* How very sweet of you. We will do that when Val feels better. I know you were worried about him.

JUNIOR   *[Sign]* We care about Val. Please tell us everything about him. We need to get to know him.

HUMPHREY   *[Sign]* Really, what would you like to know about him?

JUNIOR   *[Sign]* Hmmm. Everything, including his birth.

HUMPHREY   *[Sign]* His birth?

JUNIOR   *[Sign]* Yes, we would love to hear that.

HUMPHREY   *(In tears) [Sign]* I am afraid I can't tell you.

The kids gasp.

TRACI   *[Sign]* Why not?

HUMPHREY   *(In tears) [Sign]* It will make you cry, it is a sad story.

TRACI   *[Sign]* Come on, we accept who he is. He is our friend no matter what.

JUNIOR   *[Sign]* Please tell us.

HUMPHREY   *[Sign]* Okay. Are you sure?

The students nod their heads.

HUMPHREY   *[Sign]* Matthew, please close the door.

MATTHEW   *[Sign]* Okay. *(Closes the door and sits down)*

Humphrey goes to her desk and gets tissues to give her students.

HUMPHREY   *[Sign]* You ready?

JUNIOR   *[Sign]* Wait, *(Turns to Stephen)* please listen carefully. It is not funny. It is serious.

STEPHEN   *[Sign]* Okay. I will listen. We are ready.

HUMPHREY   *[Sign]* Val was born with no ears and recessed jaws in the local hospital. The doctor didn't know what to do. He was sent to Duke Hospital after his birth. His parents refused to give up on him. They asked the doctor if they could take Val home. The doctors decided to get a personal nurse who stayed with the family and she taught them to take care of Val. He was born deaf. After two months, he finally went home and met his big brother. He was forced to learn how to walk at age 4. His full name is Billie Fallon Melvin III, his parents decided to call him Val at six weeks old. I am glad that he has a caring and loving family.

JUNIOR   *(In tears)* *[Sign]* Wow. It is a very sad story, but I am glad he is alright. How did you know about that?

HUMPHREY   *[Sign]* His mother wrote me a letter about his birth. It brought me to tears. Do you believe it?

TRACI   *[Sign]* Yes, I believe you. Val will always be my friend no matter what. I guess I better move back to where I sat next to Val on the first day of school.

HUMPHREY	*[Sign]* How very sweet. You can move next to Val.
CAROLINA	*[Sign]* Humphrey, may I ask you a question?
HUMPHREY	*[Sign]* Yes, what is it?
CAROLINA	*[Sign]* How did his brother feel when he saw Val in the hospital?
HUMPHREY	*[Sign]* He was too young to understand. He was just three years old. He was so excited to meet Val when he got home from the hospital. He still loves him no matter what.
CAROLINA	*[Sign]* I understand. We have to be nice to him.
TRACI	*[Sign]* Stephen what about you, do you believe Humphrey?
STEPHEN	*[Sign]* I don't know what to say. I was scared to see what happened to Val. I felt bad.
JUNIOR	*[Sign]* Because you treated him badly?
STEPHEN	*[Sign]* Humphrey, when does Val come back from the infirmary? I want to tell him how sorry I am.
HUMPHREY	*[Sign]* That's nice. He has to rest after having a hard time swallowing. I am sure that he will be alright.
CINDY	*[Sign]* We need a sign name for Val. I am tired of fingerspelling his name. Can you help us think of one?
HUMPHREY	*[Sign]* I will help all of you if you accept Val

as your friend.

The students look at each other and nod their heads.

HUMPHREY   *[Sign]* Thanks. I got it!

TRACI   *[Sign]* What is it?

HUMPHREY   *[Sign] (V sign circle)* that's a sign name for Val.

TRACI   *[Sign]* I like that. I am sure he will like it.

The kids agree.

HUMPHREY   *[Sign]* Please don't tell Val about his sign
                    name until tomorrow morning. He will be
                    surprised.

Humphrey leaves the classroom and stops to see Cole in her office.

COLE   *[Voice]* Hey, Humphrey, I heard about what
                    happened to Val. I am very worried about
                    him.

HUMPHREY   *[Voice]* He is alright now. I am going to
                    check on him in infirmary.

COLE   *[Voice]* How sweet, you care about him.

HUMPHREY   *[Voice]* Yes, he is very special to me. I am
                    worried about his parents finding out what
                    happened.

COLE   *[Voice]* Simmons didn't call them?

HUMPHREY   *[Voice]* No. I asked her not to call them. But
                    she asked Mr. Melvin to come with his wife
                    to pick Val up, so we can discuss it in her
                    office.

COLE   *[Voice]* Okay, that's why I am worried. I
                    don't want to lose him. We need to pray for

                              them to let Val stay here.

HUMPHREY   *[Voice]* Thanks. I want you to pick Val up in
                  the infirmary when he feels better. Okay? I
                  better check on him.

COLE   *[Voice]* Okay, wait.

HUMPHREY   *[Voice]* Yes, Cole?

COLE   *[Voice]* How do your students feel?

HUMPHREY   *[Voice]* They were very scared and worried.
                  They asked me to tell them about Val's
                  birth. They were stunned. They finally accept
                  Val.

COLE   *[Voice]* Wow. That's amazing. I think you did
                  the right thing.

HUMPHREY   *[Voice]* Thanks Cole. That's what I want to
                  do for Val.

COLE   *[Voice]* Wait, Humphrey.

HUMPHREY   *[Voice]* Yes?

COLE   *(Gives the sock monkey to Humphrey) [Voice]*
                  Here is Val's sock monkey. Please take it to
                  him so he will be comfortable.

HUMPHREY   *(Holds the sock monkey) [Voice]* Okay, I will
                  take it to him. Thanks, again.

Humphrey goes to the infirmary to check on Val but he is still sleeping.

JEAN   *[Voice]* I know you are here to see Val, but he
                  is still sleeping.

HUMPHREY   *[Voice]* Yes. I want to check on how he is
                  doing. I have his sock monkey. He needs it.

JEAN   *[Voice]* Sure, I will let you go in the room to see him.

HUMPHREY   *(Puts the sock monkey on to the bed)* *[Voice]* Val, I am sure you will be alright. You will have friends soon. I don't want to lose you. I pray that your parents will let you stay here after finding out. I want to say how much I love you.

Humphrey cries.

JEAN   *[Voice]* Humphrey, you okay?

HUMPHREY   *[Voice]* Yes. I wanted to take him home and take care of him, but Simmons wouldn't let me do that. Please let me know how Val is doing.

JEAN   *[Voice]* Okay, please relax when you get home.

Humphrey smiles and kisses Val's cheek. She waves goodbye to Jean and leaves.

In the girls' dorm, the girls are playing, but Traci doesn't feel like it because she's still thinking about Val.

THE GIRL'S HOUSEPARENT   *[Sign]* You okay, Traci?

TRACI   *[Sign]* Yes. I am fine.

THE GIRL'S HOUSEPARENT   *[Sign]* I thought you wanted to play with the other girls?

TRACI   *[Sign]* I need to be alone for now.

THE GIRL'S HOUSEPARENT   *[Sign]* Okay, alright.

CINDY   *[Sign]* Traci, I know it is about Val. I am still thinking about him too.

CAROLINA   *[Sign]* Me too. We will talk to him when he
                    gets here.

TRACI   *[Sign]* And we will make him very happy. I
                    hope the boys feel the same way.

CINDY   *[Sign]* Who?

TRACI   *[Sign]* Stephen, Junior, and Matthew.

*At the Eagles Hall Playground, the boys play outside. Junior stands alone
thinking about Val.*

JUNIOR   *[Sign]* I don't feel like playing outside.

MATTHEW   *[Sign]* Neither do I.

STEPHEN   *[Sign]* Hey, want to play ball with me?

JUNIOR   *[Sign]* No, I don't want to play, thanks.

MATTHEW   *[Sign]* I don't feel like it.

STEPHEN   *[Sign]* Why are the two of you sitting around
                    thinking about Val?

JUNIOR   *[Sign]* Yes, we are thinking about him. What
                    about you?

STEPHEN   *[Sign]* He is still in the infirmary. He needs
                    rest for now. Come play with me.

MATTHEW   *[Sign]* Junior is right. We have to wait until
                    Val gets back. He needs friends.

JUNIOR   *[Sign]* You said you accept Val as your
                    friend. Right?

STEPHEN   *[Sign]* You are right. I guess I will join you.

JUNIOR   *[Sign]* Yeah. We will wait for Val.

In Cole's office, she gets a call from Val's mother.

COLE	*[Voice]* Hello this is Thelma Cole who is this?
BETTY	*[Voice]* Hello Cole! This is Mrs. Melvin. How is my son doing? I hope he is enjoying school.
COLE	*(Clears her throat) [Voice]* He is doing alright. I heard Humphrey invited him to her house for supper with her and her family. He had a great time.
BETTY	*[Voice]* It sounded great. I am glad she did. Has he made friends yet?
COLE	*[Voice]* Umm, he is working on making friends.
BETTY	*[Voice]* It is great to hear! Please send Val my love. Thanks, see you Friday.
COLE	*[Voice]* Sure no problem, I will see you then. Bye.
	(Hangs up feeling guilty) [Voice] I can't believe I lied to her again.

The next morning, the students are in the classroom with Mrs. Humphrey, but Val is not there.

HUMPHREY	*[Sign]* Junior, have you seen Val yet? I need to know what happened.
JUNIOR	*[Sign]* I saw him at breakfast. Val is acting strange and quiet. I don't know what's wrong with him.
HUMPHREY	*[Sign]* I better go and check on him.

DAWSON   *(Shows up)* *[Voice]* Hello, Humphrey, I want you to know Val is at the dorm. Simmons and Cole are there with him. He is acting strange. I think he needs you now. I will watch your students for you.

HUMPHREY   *[Voice to Dawson and sign to her students]* Thanks Dawson, I will be there. *(Turns to her students)* Please stay here and behave yourself for Dawson. I will be back.

TRACI   *[Sign]* What's wrong with Val? We want to talk to him and give him a big hug.

HUMPHREY   *[Sign]* I know. I will let you know how he is.

Humphrey leaves for the dorm. Meanwhile, Cole and Simmons are at the dorm with Val who sits against the wall, next to the bed. They try to get Val up, but he refuses to move. He holds his sock monkey.

SIMMONS   *[Voice]* That's it. I am going to spank him now. He is not listening to what I say.

COLE   *[Voice]* Please don't do that, I believe he is acting strange because of what happened yesterday. We need Humphrey to comfort him.

SIMMONS   *[Voice]* I know, but I just asked him to go to class. He refused to move. I need to spank him to make him obey.

HUMPHREY   *(Shows up)* *[Voice]* Simmons, please don't spank him. Let me handle him. He must be having a hard time.

SIMMONS   *[Voice]* How did you know?

HUMPHREY   *[Voice]* Look at him, he needs love and support. Let me talk to Val please.

SIMMONS   *[Voice]* Sure, okay.

HUMPHREY   *[Sign]* Val, I am here with you, please tell me
                    what's wrong with you. I won't let Simmons
                    spank you.

VAL   *(Cries) [Sign]* I thought I was going to die
                    yesterday.

HUMPHREY   *[Sign]* Oh Val, please don't say that. You are
                    lucky to be alive. Please don't think about
                    yesterday.

VAL   *[Sign]* I don't want to go to your class again.

HUMPHREY   *[Sign]* Why not?

VAL   *[Sign]* My classmates dislike me because I am
                    different. Nobody likes me.

HUMPHREY   *[Sign]* They asked me about you when you
                    were in the infirmary. They were worried
                    about you and they want to be your friends.

VAL   *[Sign]* Are you sure?

HUMPHREY   *[Sign]* Yes, come with me.

VAL   *[Sign]* Okay. I will get up if Simmons will not
                    spank me

HUMPHREY   *[Voice]* Simmons, please drop your belt so
                    Val will get up.

SIMMONS   *[Voice]* Okay, I won't spank him. *(Drops the
                    belt)*

VAL   *(Gets up) [Sign]* Thanks Simmons.

COLE   *[Voice]* Wow, you did an amazing job.

SIMMONS   *[Voice]* Good job. It is time to go to class.
                   See you later.

HUMPHREY   *[Voice to Simmons and sign to Val]* Thanks,
                   Simmons. *(Turns to Val)* Come with me, Val.

*Humphrey and Val walk in the hallway to the classroom, but Val is very
nervous about seeing his classmates. Humphrey holds his hand.*

HUMPHREY   *[Sign]* What's wrong? Your classmates are
                   waiting for you.

VAL   *[Sign]* I am too nervous to see them.

HUMPHREY   *[Sign]* Please don't worry. They want to be
                   your friends. Come with me.

VAL   *[Sign]* Okay, hold me.

HUMPHREY   *[Sign]* Okay. *(Turns to her students)* Val had a
                   hard time yesterday. He is afraid to go to
                   class. Tell him all of you want to be his
                   friends.

TRACI   *[Sign]* Val, don't be afraid. I am always very
                   nice. Let me hug you. *(Hugs Val)* Feel better?

VAL   *[Sign]* Aww. Thanks, Traci. What about the
                   others?

TRACI   *[Sign]* Hey everyone, please go hug Val and
                   tell him you are his friends.

CAROLINA   *[Sign]* We have a surprise for you. You have
                   a sign name.

VAL   *[Sign]* Really? What is it?

CAROLINA   *[Sign]* Please watch us sign your name.

The students make a "V" in a circle as Humphrey and Val look on.

HUMPHREY   *[Sign]* Val, what do you think?

VAL   *[Sign]* I love it! Thanks so much!

HUMPHREY   *[Sign]* Thanks so much for making him very
             happy. Give him a hug and make him feel
             welcome here.

Val's classmates greet and hug him as Humphrey looks at them. Simmons shows up and finds the students hugging each other. Mrs. Humphrey tell Simmons it is a miracle. Later, when the students are done with language work, Humphrey has Val stay with her.

HUMPHREY   *[Sign]* You all did well. I am proud of all of
             you. It is time for recess. Val, you need to stay
             here.

VAL   *[Sign]* Am I bad?

HUMPHREY   *[Sign]* No, I have something for you to eat.

JUNIOR   *[Sign]* We want him to play hide and seek. Why
             do you want him to stay here?

HUMPHREY   *[Sign]* I made oatmeal for him. He needs to eat
             soft foods. I hope you all understand.

TRACI   *[Sign]* I understand. You sound like you are his
             mother.

HUMPHREY   *[Sign]* I know. It is time to go to recess. Don't
             worry about Val. I will take care of him.

The kids leave for recess and Humphrey goes to the Teacher's Lounge and pours water into the oatmeal as Val looks on. Simmons comes in and looks at them.

SIMMONS   *[Voice]* Humphrey, what are you doing with
             Val?

HUMPHREY   *[Voice to Simmons and sign to Val]* I made some oatmeal for him. *(Turns to Val)* How do you like oatmeal?

VAL   *[Sign]* Good, I love it. I need milk too.

HUMPHREY   *[Sign]* Okay, I will get it as soon as I finish talking with Simmons.

SIMMONS   *[Voice]* I understand why. It is very nice of you to be concerned. We have to talk with his parents. They are on the way now.

HUMPHREY   *[Voice]* You want me there in your office?

SIMMONS   *[Voice]* Yes, you were a witness when Val choked on the sausage. I won't tell them until they get here.

HUMPHREY   *[Voice]* That's what I am worried about.

VAL   *[Sign]* It is hot. I need milk now.

HUMPHREY   *[Sign]* Take it easy. Be patient.

SIMMONS   *[Voice]* I feel the same way you do. We have to explain everything to them. I hope they won't be angry.

HUMPHREY   *[Voice]* Me too. Can you watch Val while I get milk?

SIMMONS   *[Voice]* Sure, go on. I need to talk to Val.

HUMPHREY   *[Voice to Simmons sign to Val]* Sure, thanks. Val, I will get milk now. *(She leaves)*

SIMMONS   *[Sign]* Hello Val. How do you feel?

VAL   *[Sign]* I am better. My classmates want to be friends with me. I am very happy.

SIMMONS	*[Sign]* That's wonderful. You can tell your parents that you finally made friends. They will be happy to hear. They are on the way now.
VAL	*[Sign]* Okay. Do they know?
SIMMONS	*[Sign]* Not yet. I want to say I am so sorry I gave you a hard time. I tried to help you.
VAL	*[Sign]* It is okay. You are forgiven.
SIMMONS	*[Sign]* Thank you. Can I give you a hug? I am worried.
VAL	*[Sign]* Everyone is worried. That's why they hugged me.
SIMMONS	*[Sign]* We care about you. Can I hug you?
VAL	*[Sign]* Come on, but don't spill my oatmeal.
SIMMONS	*[Sign]* You get up so I can hug you.

Val gets up and Simmons hugs him as Humphrey looks at them and smiles.

They are in Humphrey's classroom and Val is acting strange; he is tears as Traci looks at him.

TRACI	*[Sign]* You okay?
VAL	*[Sign]* No.
TRACI	*[Sign]* What's wrong?
VAL	*[Sign]* My mama and papa will be mad.
TRACI	*(Raises her hand) [Sign]* Humphrey?
HUMPHREY	*[Sign]* Yes, Traci what's wrong?
TRACI	*[Sign]* It is Val. He looks very upset about his parents.

HUMPHREY	*[Sign]* Val, please tell me what's wrong.
VAL	*(Cries) [Sign]* They will get mad when they find out what happened.
HUMPHREY	*(Comforts Val) [Sign]* Please don't worry. Simmons and I will explain everything to them. It will be alright.
VAL	*[Sign]* What if they pull me out of school?
HUMPHREY	*[Sign]* Please relax. We will tell them we will take care of you. *(Hugs him)* Take it easy, I am here with you.
JUNIOR	*[Sign]* What's wrong?
TRACI	*[Sign]* He is worried that Simmons and Humphrey will tell his parents about what happened.
STEPHEN	*[Sign]* How we treated him badly?
JUNIOR	*[Sign]* No, about swallowing the sausage.

Betty arrives at Eagles Hall and sees Mrs. Cole at her desk. Cole looks around.

BETTY	*[Voice]* Hello Mrs. Cole. I am here.
COLE	*[Voice]* Hello, Mrs. Melvin. Happy to see you. Where is your husband? Simmons needed you to bring him.
BETTY	*[Voice]* I am so sorry, but something has happened. His work needed him because his coworker is out.
COLE	*[Voice]* Alright, let me call Simmons.
BETTY	*[Voice]* Okay. She called me and told me to come to her office for a meeting about Val. Is

he in trouble?

SIMMONS   *(Shows up and walks in) [Voice]* Hello Mrs.
Melvin. No, Val is not in trouble. Your
husband is not here with you?

BETTY   *[Voice]* I am so sorry. He has to work because
his coworker is sick. Is it okay to discuss it
with me? I will tell him when I get home.

SIMMONS   *[Voice]* Alright, Mrs. Melvin, please stay in the
lobby until the class is finished. I will call you.

COLE   *[Voice]* I will keep her company. Would you
care for coffee?

BETTY   *[Voice]* Thanks Cole.

Meanwhile the students are doing math work.

VAL   *(Gives his math paper to Humphrey) [Sign]* I am
finished. You can check it.

HUMPHREY   *(Looks at the paper) [Sign]* Thanks, let me see it.

Val laughs.

HUMPHREY   *[Sign]* What is funny?

VAL   *[Sign]* Math is fun. I love it.

HUMPHREY   *[Sign]* It is the first time I've see you laugh. It is
very nice. Let me check your paper.

HUMPHREY   *[Sign]* You did a great job. I will put a star on
it.

VAL   *[Sign]* I did it! I did it!

HUMPHREY   *[Sign]* Val got a 100 on math. Please clap for
him.

The students raise their hands and clap which cheers Val up. He smiles.

VAL   *[Sign]* Thank you so much!

After class, Val is nervous about seeing his parents.

HUMPHREY   *[Sign]* Class is dismissed. It is time to go home. Have a great weekend. *(The students leave)*

VAL   *[Sign]* Can I stay here longer?

HUMPHREY   *[Sign]* Why?

VAL   *[Sign]* I am very nervous about seeing mama and papa.

HUMPHREY   *[Sign]* They are not mad. They love you no matter what.

VAL   *[Sign]* But you and Simmons will tell them everything.

HUMPHREY   *[Sign]* Please take it easy. It will be alright. They are waiting for you.

Humphrey and Val go to the middle of Eagles Hall where they meet Simmons and Val's mother.

VAL   *[Sign]* Mama, where is papa?

BETTY   *[Sign]* He can't make it; he has to work.

VAL   *[Sign]* Okay.

BETTY   *[Sign]* Where's my hug?

HUMPHREY   *[Sign]* Come on, please give her a big hug.

VAL   *(Hugs his mama) [Sign]* Mama, I missed you. I got a 100 in Math.

BETTY   *[Sign]* Really? Wow! I am proud of you.

VAL	*[Sign]* Humphrey helped me a lot.
BETTY	*[Voice]* Thanks so much Humphrey. Did Val have a great time at your place for supper?
HUMPHREY	*[Voice]* Yes, he did.
SIMMONS	*[Voice]* It is time for our meeting in my office. Cole, keep Val company.
VAL	*[Sign]* I need to get my suitcase.
COLE	*[Sign]* It is in my office. Come on Val.
VAL	*[Sign]* Mama, I will see you later. *(He and Cole go to her office)*
HUMPHREY	*[Voice]* Simmons, may I have a minute with you?
SIMMONS	*[Voice]* Sure, but Mrs. Melvin is with us.
BETTY	*[Voice]* Excuse me, I need to go to restroom. I will be back soon.
SIMMONS	*[Voice]* Sure, take your time.
HUMPHREY	*[Voice]* It is not a good time to talk to her because her husband is not here. It will be very difficult.
SIMMONS	*[Voice]* I know, but we will take care of everything.
HUMPHREY	*[Voice]* She was very scared of losing Val after his birth. She refused to give up on him.
SIMMONS	*[Voice]* It is very different. Val is doing fine.
BETTY	*[Voice]* I am back. I am ready for the meeting.

SIMMONS   *[Voice]* Good, Mrs. Melvin, let's go to my
                 office.

They go to Simmons' office.

BETTY   *[Voice]* Hold up, Simmons, I want to say Mrs.
                 Humphrey thanks so much for inviting Val to
                 your house. Mr. Melvin and I appreciated
                 what you did for my son.

HUMPHREY   *[Voice]* Aww, Mrs. Melvin, I enjoyed having
                 him with us.

BETTY   *[Voice]* What did your husband and your sons
                 think about him?

HUMPHREY   *[Voice]* They think he is very special. Guess
                 what? Val has a sign name for Alan.

BETTY   *[Voice]* Really? Show it to me.

HUMPHREY   *[Voice]* Wait until the meeting is over.

SIMMONS   *[Voice]* Humphrey, Mrs. Melvin, we are not
                 here to discuss inviting Val to your place. We
                 need to discuss something different.

BETTY   *[Voice]* I am so sorry. I wanted to ask how it
                 went. What is the problem with Val? Did he
                 behave badly or refuse to eat?

SIMMONS   *[Voice]* We need to discuss what happened at
                 lunch yesterday.

BETTY   *[Voice]* Okay, tell me now.

SIMMONS   *[Voice]* Humphrey, tell her what Val was
                 eating for lunch.

HUMPHREY   *[Voice]* We were having greens, corn, and
                 sausage.

BETTY	*[Voice]* Sausage? It is a hard food for him to chew. Did you cut it before he ate?
HUMPHREY	*[Voice]* Simmons, tell her, I don't think I can.
SIMMONS	*[Voice]* But you are the witness.
BETTY	*[Voice]* Pardon me, tell me, did you cut the food for Val or not?
HUMPHREY	*[Voice]* I hate to say this, but I forgot to cut it.
BETTY	*[Voice]* You let him eat it?
HUMPHREY	*[Voice]* Yes...
BETTY	*[Voice]* And?
HUMPHREY	*[Voice]* I don't want you to get mad at me. I know you wanted me to cut the food before he eats.
BETTY	*[Voice]* Oh no, don't tell me he tried to swallow the sausage without chewing?
HUMPHREY	*[Voice]* That's what I am afraid to say.
BETTY	*(Gets upset)* *[Voice]* That's it, bye! *(She leaves)*

Betty rushes to Cole's office.

COLE	*[Voice]* I know you are worried, but everything is alright.
BETTY	*(Shows up and grabs Val's arm)* *[Sign]* Val, it is time to go home.
VAL	*[Sign]* Are you mad?
COLE	*[Voice]* Wait a minute, I need to talk to you.
BETTY	*[Voice]* Sorry, we have to go home. Goodbye!

VAL   *[Sign]* Can I say goodbye to Mrs. Humphrey?

BETTY   *[Sign]* No, we better go home now.

Humphrey rushes outside and tries to stop Mrs. Melvin from leaving.

HUMPHREY   *[Voice]* Wait for me!

Betty ignores her. They leave for home and Humphrey is in tears.

HUMPHREY   *(Cries) [Voice]* Oh no! It is my fault! I lost him!

SIMMONS   *[Voice]* He will be back on Sunday.

HUMPHREY   *[Voice]* She is angry at me. I tried to explain what happened, but she refused to listen to me.

SIMMONS   *[Voice]* Don't worry, she will change her mind. Mr. Melvin will talk with her. Val will be back.

COLE   *[Voice]* I hope so.

HUMPHREY   *[Voice]* I can't help it. I love him.

SIMMONS   *[Voice]* Take it easy. Everything will be fine.

On Monday morning all of the students are in the classroom, except for Val. Humphrey wonders where he is.

HUMPHREY   *[Sign]* Good morning students. Did Val come yesterday?

JUNIOR   *[Sign]* I didn't see him come here.

HUMPHREY   *[Sign]* Oh no, I better go to see Simmons. I will be back.

Humphrey goes to the office and knocks on the door.

HUMPHREY   *[Voice]* Simmons, Val is not here. I am worried about him.

SIMMONS   *[Voice]* He didn't come back yesterday?

HUMPHREY   *[Voice]* That's right. Junior told me that.

SIMMONS   *[Voice]* We better check with Cole to see if she has heard from his parents.

Humphrey and Simmons go to Cole's office.

HUMPHREY   *[Voice]* Hello Cole. Have you seen or heard from Val and his parents? He is not in my class.

COLE   *[Voice]* I am so sorry, I haven't heard from them since I saw Val and his mother last Friday. I tried to call them, but no one answered.

SIMMONS   *[Voice]* Well, try to call them now.

COLE   *[Voice]* Okay. *(Dials the number)* It is ringing.

HUMPHREY   *[Voice]* Come on Melvin.

SIMMONS   *[Voice]* Humphrey! You worry too much!

HUMPHREY   *[Voice]* I can't help it. I care about that boy.

COLE   *[Voice]* I am afraid that no one answered. What should we do?

SIMMONS   *[Voice]* Well, we better wait. Humphrey, go back to your classroom. The students are waiting for you.

HUMPHREY   *[Voice]* Okay, well, see you later.

Humphrey is upset as she goes back to the classroom to teach the students.

HUMPHREY	*[Sign]* Kids, I am going to teach you about nouns, verbs, and adjectives.
TRACI	*[Sign]* I know why you are very sad. It is Val.
HUMPHREY	*[Sign]* I know, but I have to be strong so I can teach you the lesson. Please don't talk about him. Let him go.
JUNIOR	*[Sign]* Why? We still think of Val.
HUMPHREY	*[Sign]* I know how you feel, but all of you have to be positive. Let's focus on our lesson.
KATHY	*(Raises her hand) [Sign]* Humphrey, can I tell you something?
HUMPHREY	*[Sign]* Kathy, yes, what is it?
KATHY	*[Sign]* Val is still our friend no matter what.
HUMPHREY	*[Sign]* Kathy, I understand, but please don't talk about him now. He might come soon.
VAL	*(Shows up with a box of Quik to make chocolate milk) [Sign]* Hello Humphrey I am back.
HUMPHREY	*(Cries and hugs him) [Sign]* Val, am I very happy to see you. Are your parents here?
VAL	*[Sign]* Yes, they want to talk to you now.
SIMMONS	*[Sign]* Humphrey, I found someone to watch the kids while his parents meet us in my office.
HUMPHREY	*[Voice]* Are they angry?
SIMMONS	*[Voice]* Not anymore. They are here to discuss what Val can eat. Come with me.

HUMPHREY   *[Voice to Simmons and sign to students]* Okay,
              thanks. *(Turns to her students)* Please behave
              yourselves; I will be back after the meeting.

The kids are excited and hug him as Val shows them the Quik box.

BETTY   *(Hugs Humphrey)* *[Sign]* Mrs. Humphrey, I am
              so sorry I yelled at you last Friday. I was very
              scared. My husband said you took good care
              of Val. Please forgive me.

HUMPHREY   *(Smiles)* *[Voice]* Mrs. Melvin, it is okay, you are
              forgiven. I understand how you feel. I was
              scared too. I am glad you brought Val back.

SIMMONS   *[Voice]* Mr. Melvin, I am glad you and Mrs.
              Melvin came to my office to discuss this. Are
              we ready?

FALLON   *[Voice]* We have to wait for Cole to come. I
              need her here because we have a list of food
              that Val can and can't eat.

COLE   *(Comes into Simmons' office)* *[Voice]* Hello
              everyone. Here I am.

FALLON   *[Voice]* Miss Simmons, we are ready for a
              discussion. You can explain what happened
              to me. I know my wife was so scared. I am so
              sorry I didn't make it because my work
              needed me. I took a day off so I could be
              here today.

SIMMONS   *[Voice]* Mr. Melvin, I understand, I am glad
              you are here. Last Friday was not easy to
              explain to your wife alone.

FALLON   *[Voice]* I know what you mean. I comforted
              her when they arrived home. You can explain
              everything to me.

SIMMONS	*[Voice]* Okay, Val was eating the sausage and started choking, so we got two men to take him to the infirmary. Humphrey asked them to use the suction machine which helped get the sausage out of his mouth. He was able to breath and we had him rest after that.
BETTY	*[Voice]* Humphrey, you saved our son's life.
HUMPHREY	*[Voice]* No, the nurse did.
BETTY	*[Voice]* You told them to use the suction machine to help Val breathe. You saved his life.
HUMPHREY	*[Voice]* Really, did I do that?
FALLON	*[Voice]* That's right. Thanks so much for saving his life.
BETTY	*[Voice]* You did the right thing. I am glad you went to the infirmary with him. I know you were very worried.
HUMPHREY	*[Voice]* I was very scared to see him choking. I am glad he is alright. I will take care of him for you.
BETTY	*[Voice]* Yes, my husband and I trust you.
HUMPHREY	*[Voice]* Thanks so much. I appreciate it.
SIMMONS	*[Voice]* It is wonderful news that you have decided to give us another chance to keep Val here. What would you like us to do with the food for Val?
FALLON	*[Voice]* Betty and I talked about that. She was working on the list of food that Val can and cannot eat.

BETTY	*[Voice]* Here it is. We want you to give it to the dietary staff and tell them what to do.
FALLON	*[Voice]* Talk to them about Val's recessed jaws and his inability to chew.
SIMMONS	*[Voice]* That sounds like a great idea. I will be glad to do that. Thanks so much.
FALLON	*[Voice]* Then the problem is solved. Any questions?
SIMMONS	*[Voice]* Well, I need to ask you a question. Can Val eat sausage again?
FALLON AND BETTY	*[Voice]* No way.
SIMMONS	*[Voice]* Good answer. The meeting is over. Thanks so much for coming over here. I appreciate you giving us another chance.
BETTY	*[Voice]* Thanks Miss Simmons. May we see Val before we leave?
HUMPHREY	*[Voice]* Sure, come with me.

They go to the classroom.

BETTY	*[Voice]* Humphrey, Val kept talking about you and his classmates. He wants to stay here.
HUMPHREY	*[Voice]* Wow, that's wonderful. What did he say?
BETTY	*[Voice]* He said he made friends and he is lucky to have people who love him. I was surprised. Val got his sign name; I love it.
FALLON	*[Voice]* Look at him, he has friends in the class.

HUMPHREY	*[Voice]* Yes, it is a miracle. I am glad everything is alright.
BETTY	*[Voice]* Thanks to you, he is happy here. Alan likes Val's sign name for him. Can I give him a goodbye hug before we leave?
HUMPHREY	*[Voice]* Great to hear! Help yourself.
VAL	*[Sign]* Are you going home now?
BETTY	*[Sign]* Yes, our meeting is over. We need to go home. I want to see you be happy here.
VAL	*[Sign]* I am very happy here. I have friends here.
BETTY	*[Sign]* It is great to hear. Please listen to what Humphrey says. Love you, see you Friday
FALLON	*[Sign]* Proud of you, son. Love you.
VAL	*(Hugs his parents) [Sign]* I love you. See you Friday.
BETTY	*[Sign]* Bye, sweetheart!
VAL	*[Sign]* Mama?
BETTY	*[Sign]* Yes?
VAL	*[Sign]* Don't worry about me. Humphrey will take care of me. I will be alright.
BETTY	*(Hugs her son) [Sign to Val and voice to Humphrey]* Oh, Val, yes, she will. *(Turns to Humphrey)* Please take care of our son for us. Goodbye.
HUMPHREY	*[Voice]* Mrs. Melvin, I will. Bye.
VAL	*(Hugs Humphrey) [Sign]* I have good news.

HUMPHREY	*[Sign]* Really, what is it?
VAL	*[Sign]* Mama, papa, and Alan love my sign name. Alan loves my sign name for him.
HUMPHREY	*[Sign]* That's wonderful! I am glad they love it. Now let's have class.

In the lunchroom, Val brings the Quik flavor to share with his classmates. His classmates are excited to see him with it.

HUMPHREY	*[Sign]* Kids, Val said he can share his Quik flavor. He would like to know if you want some.

The kids get excited and all of them raise their hands.

TRACI	*[Sign]* How many spoons do I put in my milk?
VAL	*[Sign]* Two spoons!
TRACI	*[Sign]* Okay.

The kids put each spoon into their milk and they drink the chocolate milk as Val looks on.

CAROLINA	*[Sign]* It is very good. I love it.
KATHY	*[Sign]* Thanks so much, Val. I like it!
MATTHEW	*(Looks at the kids from other classes) [Sign]* Why do they stare at us?
STEPHEN	*[Sign]* They are jealous of us. Ignore them.
HUMPHREY	*[Sign]* Stephen?
STEPHEN	*[Sign]* Yes?
HUMPHREY	*[Sign]* What do you want to say to Val?
STEPHEN	*[Sign]* I don't know what to say.

JUNIOR   *(Touches Stephen and whispers)* *[Sign]* Tell him thanks for the chocolate milk.

STEPHEN   *[Sign]* Oh, I forgot. I am so sorry. Val, thanks so much. I enjoyed it.

VAL   *[Sign]* You are welcome.

STEPHEN   *[Sign]* I am so sorry I treated you badly. I was wrong about you. Can we be friends?

VAL   *[Sign]* Yes, we can be friends. You are forgiven.

STEPHEN   *[Sign]* Oh, thanks, Val!

HUMPHREY   *[Sign]* Kids, I am glad you like Val's chocolate milk, but eat your lunch before it gets cold.

VAL   *[Sign]* My lunch is not here. Where is it?

HUMPHREY   *[Sign]* Here it comes. Robin fixed your food. It is soft so you can eat it.

ROBIN   *(Puts the food on the table)* *[Sign]* Hello Val, you can eat now. The food is soft.

SIMMONS   *(Comes to the table)* *[Voice]* Hello, I am here to determine if Val likes it or not.

HUMPHREY   *[Sign]* Val, eat your lunch. We want to know if you like it or not. Tell me.

VAL   *[Sign]* Okay. I see pork chops cut up. Corn and beans are soft enough for me. *(Eats his lunch)*

SIMMONS   *[Sign]* What do you think Val?

VAL   *(Thumbs up)* *[Sign]* They are very good.

ROBIN	*[Sign]* Thanks so much. We will do our best for you.
VAL	*[Sign]* Okay, no more sausages for me.
ROBIN	*[Voice]* No more sausages? He doesn't like them?
SIMMONS	*[Voice]* It is hard for him to eat. He wants you to skip sausages. His parents don't want him to eat it again.
ROBIN	*[Voice]* Got it. OK, I am glad Val likes the food.
VAL	*[Sign]* Thanks so much Robin.
ROBIN	*[Sign]* Welcome, anytime.
SIMMONS	*[Voice]* The kids look very happy. They must be nice to him.
HUMPHREY	*[Voice]* Yes. He brought Quik chocolate flavor and shared it with his classmates. It made them happy.
SIMMONS	*[Voice to Humphrey and sign to Val]* Great to hear. Val, enjoy your lunch.

Scene Eight: Teaching Val How to Express Himself

The kids play outside at the Eagles Hall Playground. They invite Val to ride on the merry-go-round. Val's shoelaces get untied and he asks Cassandra to tie them. She ties his shoes and wonders why he has not learned how to do it himself. She walks to Mrs. Humphrey.

CASSANDRA	*[Sign]* I need to talk to you about Val. I actually like him, but he is lazy.

HUMPHREY	*[Sign]* Pardon me, why are you calling him lazy?
CASSANDRA	*[Sign]* I am so sorry, I didn't mean it like that. His shoelaces were untied and he asked me to tie them. I think he should have to do it himself.
HUMPHREY	*[Sign]* I know what you mean. I think it is time for him to learn himself.
CASSANDRA	*[Sign]* Great! When will you teach him?
HUMPHREY	*[Sign]* After class.

The kids do math work in the classroom. Class is dismissed, but as the other kids leave, Humphrey asks Val to stay with her.

HUMPHREY	*[Sign]* Kids, class is dismissed; it is time to get going to the dorm. See all of you tomorrow, don't forget your homework.
KIDS	*(Wave at Humphrey and leave) [Sign]* Okay.
HUMPHREY	*[Sign]* Val, please stay here.
VAL	*[Sign]* Okay, why?
HUMPHREY	*[Sign]* I have an important lesson to teach you.
VAL	*[Sign]* Okay, what is it?
HUMPHREY	*[Sign]* It is time for you to tie your shoes yourself.
VAL	*[Sign]* I don't know how to do it. You can tie them.
HUMPHREY	*[Sign]* Well, okay, please watch me tie your shoes so you can learn how.

VAL	*[Sign]* Okay.
HUMPHREY	*[Sign]* I am going to untie your shoes now.
VAL	*(Gets upset) [Sign]* Why?
HUMPHREY	*[Sign]* You have to tie your shoes yourself; you are a big boy like Junior.
VAL	*[Sign]* Okay, I am going to do it myself.

Val tries to tie, but he loses his temper when he doesn't do it well.

VAL	*(Cries) [Sign]* I am very sorry; I can't do it.
HUMPHREY	*[Sign]* Okay, take it easy. *(Looks at a picture of Alan in a project for Val's family)* Do you want to be a big boy like your brother?
VAL	*[Sign]* Yes, I want to.
HUMPHREY	*[Sign]* Please think about him while you are tying your shoes.
VAL	*[Sign]* Okay. *(Tries to tie his shoes)* Humphrey, I did it! I did it!
HUMPHREY	*(Hugs Val) [Sign]* Good boy! You did an amazing job!
VAL	*[Sign]* It is easy. Can I do it again?
HUMPHREY	*[Sign]* Sure, go on.
VAL	*[Sign]* I did it again, I am a big boy.
HUMPHREY	*[Sign]* That's right. You can do everything yourself.
VAL	*[Sign]* Like what?
HUMPHREY	*[Sign]* Getting dressed, bathing, making your

bed, and brushing your teeth like Alan does.

VAL	*[Sign]* Okay, I will try my best.
HUMPHREY	*[Sign]* Please don't give up, okay?
VAL	*[Sign]* Okay, I won't.

After supper, Val walks in the hallway and passes Cole's office as Mrs. Cole looks at him.

COLE	*[Sign]* Val, where are you going? To the infirmary?
VAL	*[Sign]* That's right. I know which way to go.
COLE	*[Sign]* Are you sure you don't need me to go with you?
VAL	*[Sign]* I don't want to hurt your feelings, but I know how to get there. I am a big boy. Thanks so much.
COLE	*(Smiles)* *[Sign]* I understand. Be careful, it is dark.

Val goes to the infirmary, Jean Barnes is surprised to see him arrive alone.

JEAN	*[Sign]* Hello Val, you came here yourself?
VAL	*[Sign]* Yes, I knew where to go. I am a big boy.
JEAN	*[Sign]* Really? Does Mrs. Cole know that?
VAL	*[Sign]* Yes, she knows I am a big boy. I am ready for the suction machine.
JEAN	*[Sign]* Sure, come on.

VAL	*[Sign]* After that, I will brush my teeth myself.
JEAN	*[Sign]* Are you sure you can do it?
VAL	*[Sign]* Yes, I am a big boy.

Jean Barnes laughs and inserts Val's trach to clean. Val begins to brush his teeth himself as Jean watches him.

That night, Miss Bass checks on the boys at the shower. Val grabs the cloth from Miss Bass' hand. He washes himself and pours water over his head to rinse the shampoo. Miss Bass is in tears. She tells him she is proud of him.

In the morning, Miss Bass is very surprised to see Val dress himself. Miss Bass asks him if she can brush his hair. Val tells her he can do it himself. He makes the bed like the other kids do. Miss Bass runs to Cole's office and tells her the good news.

In the classroom, Val tells his classmates that he can do everything like they do. They raise their hands and congratulate him as Humphrey looks on.

Later, on Friday afternoon, the kids get ready to go home. Humphrey asks Val to stay for a while.

VAL	*[Sign]* Did I do something wrong?
HUMPHREY	*[Sign]* No, you did well. I want to say I am proud of you for doing everything yourself.
VAL	*[Sign]* Thanks so much, I can't wait to tell Mama and Papa.
HUMPHREY	*[Sign]* No, you don't have to tell them. Just show them you can do everything yourself and they will be surprised.
VAL	*[Sign]* Sure, do you think they will be proud of me?
HUMPHREY	*[Sign]* Yes. They will always be proud. Your

mama is waiting for you. Have a great
weekend and see you Monday.

VAL   *(Hugs her) [Sign]* Okay, thanks for everything
                       again. See you on Monday.

*Val and his mother leave to go home as Cole looks on. Humphrey walks
past her office.*

HUMPHREY   *[Voice]* Hey Cole, have a great weekend.

COLE   *[Voice]* You too. Wait, did you tell Mrs. Melvin
                       about Val doing everything himself, like tying
                       his shoes and going to the infirmary himself?

HUMPHREY   *[Voice]* No, he will surprise them when he is at
                       home this weekend. I know they will be
                       excited.

COLE   *[Voice]* What if Mrs. Melvin wants to see you
                       on Sunday?

HUMPHREY   *[Voice]* If they want to see me, they can come
                       to my place. I feel very close to Val, I love
                       him.

COLE   *[Voice]* You love him? That's sweet of you.
                       Does he know you love him?

HUMPHREY   *[Voice]* Not yet. I decided to wait for him to
                       tell me he loves me. Then I will tell him the
                       same thing.

COLE   *[Voice]* I understand. Please let me know when
                       he tells you that. Have a good weekend.

HUMPHREY   *[Voice]* You too, bye

*On Monday afternoon, Val writes a letter to his parents as Humphrey looks
on. Val asks her if she can get another paper for him to write. After class,
Humphrey finds a note from Val. It says "I love you." Humphrey cries and*

rushes to the dorm to look for Val. She finds him outside. She pulls him away and goes to Cole's office.

COLE	*[Voice]* Hello Humphrey, what are you doing with Val? Is he in trouble again?
HUMPHREY	*[Voice]* No, he told me he loves me for the first time.
COLE	*[Sign]* Really? Val, you told her you love her?
VAL	*[Sign]* Yes, I told her I love her because she is sweet and kind to me.
COLE	*[Sign to Val and voice to Humphrey]* That's wonderful. I am very happy the two of you have gotten closer. Humphrey, did you tell him you love him?
HUMPHREY	*[Voice]* I did, look at Val. He is weeping.
COLE	*[Sign]* Aww sweet, need tissues?
VAL	*[Sign]* Yes, I need them please.
COLE	*[Sign]* Here they are.
HUMPHREY	*[Voice]* My family and I would like to take him out to eat.
COLE	*[Voice]* Really, what for?
HUMPHREY	*[Voice]* As a reward for him. I already called his parents and they gave me permission.
COLE	*[Voice]* But what about Simmons?
SIMMONS	*(Is on her way home, but sees them)* *[Voice]* Hey, Humphrey, are you going to take Val somewhere?

HUMPHREY	*[Voice]* Yes, it is to reward him.
SIMMONS	*[Voice]* A reward for what?
HUMPHREY	*[Sign]* Val, tell her.
VAL	*[Sign]* I can do everything myself, like tying my shoes, brushing my teeth, going to the infirmary, and getting dressed myself. *(He ties his shoes)*
SIMMONS	*[Sign]* Wow, I am very happy for you. You can go to eat with Humphrey and her family.
VAL	*[Sign]* Thanks so much, Simmons.
HUMPHREY	*[Sign]* Come on, Val, my husband and sons are waiting for us.
VAL	*[Sign]* I can't go.
HUMPHREY	*[Sign]* Why not? I thought you wanted to go.
VAL	*[Sign]* I want to go, but I am worried my classmates will be jealous. Remember what happened last time?
HUMPHREY	*[Sign]* Yes, I explained everything to them. They understand, you don't have to worry.
VAL	*[Sign]* Okay. I feel better.

Scene Nine: A Visit from the Grandparents

On Friday, Val goes to the infirmary to be suctioned and brush his teeth. He runs into a couple he knows. Humphrey wonders why Val is staying in the infirmary for so long and goes to Miss Simmons' office.

HUMPHREY	*[Voice]* Simmons, have you seen Val? He is

not back from the infirmary.

SIMMONS   *[Voice]* Okay, I will call the nurse to see what's going on.

HUMPHREY   *(Looks at Val walking with two people) [Voice]* Here he is. He is with two people.

SIMMONS   *[Voice]* Who are they?

HUMPHREY   *[Voice]* I don't know. Let's find out.

VAL   *[Sign]* Humphrey, Grandma and Grandpa are here to see me. They found me in the infirmary.

HUMPHREY   *[Voice]* Oh, *(Turns to Simmons)* they are his grandparents.

GRANDMA   *[Voice]* We are so sorry if Val is late. We found him in the infirmary. We picked the suction machine up to take it home.

HUMPHREY   *[Voice]* Okay, does Mrs. Melvin know you are here to pick Val up?

GRANDMA   *[Voice]* Yes, my daughter doesn't feel well and she asked us to pick him up and take him home.

HUMPHREY   *[Voice]* Your daughter? Oh! You must be the parents of Mrs. Melvin, right? I am so sorry about her, I hope she will get better soon.

GRANDMA   *[Voice]* That's right. My name is Merle Woodburn and this is my husband, Maurice. I know you are Mrs. Humphrey, Betty told me so much about you. You are our grandson's teacher.

HUMPHREY	*[Voice]* Nice to meet you.
GRANDPA	*[Voice and sign]* Who is this?
VAL	*(Sign as Humphrey tells Grandpa in voice)* Miss Simmons. She is my principal.
SIMMONS	*[Voice]* That's right. Nice to meet you. You will have to stay in the lobby because class will not be over for two hours.
HUMPHREY	*[Voice to the grandparents and sign to Val]* That's right, *(Turns to Val)* it is time to go back to class and work on math.
VAL	*[Sign]* Grandma brought cookies for our class.
HUMPHREY	*[Sign]* Oh how sweet, I will come get you when the work is done.
VAL	*[Sign]* I have to go to class now. See you later.
GRANDMA	*[Sign]* Please pay attention to your teacher.
VAL	*[Sign]* Right! *(Humphrey and Val go to the classroom)*
GRANDMA	*[Voice]* Simmons, can we have milk for the kids when I give them cookies?
SIMMONS	*[Voice]* That would be nice.
GRANDMA	*[Voice]* Would you like some cookies?
SIMMONS	*[Voice]* I would love one. *(Eats cookie)* It is very good, we will go get milk soon.
GRANDMA	*[Voice]* Thanks, Simmons.

The students finish their math work. Humphrey invites Val's grandparents to come to the classroom. They bring cookies and milk to the kids. Val introduces his classmates to his grandparents. They thank his grandma for the cookies. The students leave to get ready to go home, but Val and his grandparents stay in the classroom.

GRANDMA	*[Voice]* Humphrey, thanks so much for inviting us. The students seem very nice, I am glad they enjoyed the cookies.
HUMPHREY	*[Voice]* Sure, you made them very happy. I was pleased to have you here. What would you like to do now?
GRANDMA	*[Voice]* We would like to see Val learn from you. Betty told me about that.
HUMPHREY	*[Voice]* Okay, what would you like to see?
GRANDPA	*[Voice]* Tell Val to show Grandpa how he ties his shoes.
HUMPHREY	*[Sign]* Grandpa would like to see you tie your shoes.
VAL	*[Sign]* Okay, look at me. *(Ties his shoes)* It is easy; I am a big boy like Alan.
GRANDPA	*[Sign to Val and voice to Humphrey]* Good boy, I am proud of you. *(Turns to Humphrey)* Tell Val to teach me how to sign milkshake. We will stop to get it for him.
HUMPHREY	*(Laughs) [Voice to Grandpa and sign to Val]* Okay, *(Turns to Val)* Grandpa wants you to teach him the sign for milkshake. He will get one for you soon.
VAL	*[Sign]* Aww thanks. *(Helps his grandpa sign milkshake)* Here is the sign for milkshake.

GRANDPA	*[Sign]* Thanks, Val.
VAL	*[Sign]* Humphrey, can I show them some of my papers? I got stars on them.
HUMPHREY	*[Sign]* Sure. Get them from my desk. Please find your name.
VAL	*[Sign]* Okay. *(Shows papers to Grandma and Grandpa)* I make very good grades in math.
GRANDMA	*[Voice and sign]* Wow, you are very good at math. We are proud of you. That's why we will get a milkshake.
VAL	*[Sign]* I love drinking milkshakes.
GRANDMA	*[Voice]* Humphrey, you do an amazing job teaching him.
HUMPHREY	*[Voice]* Oh, Mrs. Woodburn, thanks.
GRANDPA	*[Sign]* It is time to go home. We better go get your suitcase and get in the car.
GRANDMA	*[Sign]* Val, please give her a hug. She is the best teacher you have.
VAL	*[Sign]* Yes, she is the best. *(Hugs Humphrey)* Thanks for letting Grandma and Grandpa come here. See you on Monday, I love you.
HUMPHREY	*(Gives an apple to Val)* *[Sign]* Aww, I love you too, have a great weekend. Here is an apple for your mother, I am sure she will like it.
GRANDPA	*(Shakes Humphrey's hand)* *[Voice]* Pleasure to meet you; I am glad Val has an amazing teacher. We better go now.
GRANDMA	*(Hugs Humphrey)* *[Voice]* Humphrey, thanks

so much for teaching our grandson. He is a quick learner. Have a good weekend.

HUMPHREY   *[Voice]* Oh, thanks, tell your daughter I said to get well soon.

GRANDMA   *[Voice]* Sure, I will do that.

Val waves at Humphrey and they leave.

HUMPHREY   *[Voice]* They made my day!

Humphrey clears her desk and gets ready to go home, but Val shows up with an apple pie. She is surprised to see him put it on her desk.

HUMPHREY   *[Sign]* Val, what are you doing?

VAL   *[Sign]* I wanted to bring an apple pie to you. I thought you and your family would like it.

HUMPHREY   *[Sign]* Grandma made it?

VAL   *[Sign]* Yes.

HUMPHREY   *[Sign]* She didn't have to do that.

GRANDMA   *(Shows up) [Voice]* I want all of you to enjoy it. We are very impressed with how well Val is doing here.

VAL   *[Sign]* Please keep it.

HUMPHREY   *[Sign and voice]* Okay, thanks. My family and I will enjoy it

VAL   *(Hugs Humphrey) [Sign]* See you on Monday, bye.

HUMPHREY   *[Voice]* Mrs. Woodburn?

GRANDMA   *[Voice]* Yes, dear?

HUMPHREY	*[Voice]* Can I give you a hug? I want to say thank you for the apple pie.
GRANDMA	*[Voice]* Yes, hug me now.
HUMPHREY	*(Hugs Grandma as Val looks on) [Voice]* I am glad you two came here. You are very sweet!
GRANDMA	*[Voice to Humphrey and sign to Val]* You too. Enjoy the apple pie. *(Turns to Val)* It is time to go get a milkshake and then go home.
VAL	*[Sign]* Okay. *(Turns to Mrs. Humphrey)* Hope you and your family enjoy the pie.

They leave as Humphrey weeps.

HUMPHREY	*[Voice]* They made my day very special!

On Monday morning, the students write letters to their parents, but Val writes a letter to his grandparents. He asks Humphrey for help.

VAL	*[Sign]* Humphrey, can I write a letter to Grandpa and Grandma? I want to thank them for coming.
HUMPHREY	*[Sign]* It sounds like a good idea, you can.
VAL	*[Sign]* Thanks, I need your help.
HUMPHREY	*[Sign]* Sure. What do you want me to do?
VAL	*[Sign]* Can I write a note about you?
HUMPHREY	*[Sign]* I don't understand, what are you talking about?
VAL	*[Sign]* I want to write how you and your family enjoyed the apple pie Grandma made.
HUMPHREY	*[Sign]* Thanks, but I will write them a thank you note. You can say thanks for visiting

here, that's all.

VAL   *[Sign]* Sure, do you have their address?

HUMPHREY   *[Sign]* Don't worry, Cole will get us their
                       address. Thanks for asking. They will be glad
                       to hear from you.

VAL   *(Smiles) [Sign]* Okay, thanks.

*They finish writing their letters and Humphrey gets the address for the
Woodburns. Grandpa and Grandma get the letter and read it. It makes
them smile.*

*One day the students take a spelling test while Humphrey is at her desk.
Traci notices Val's wet pants and she taps Val.*

TRACI   *[Sign]* I hate to say something, but your pants
                       are wet.

VAL   *[Sign]* Oh no.

TRACI   *[Sign]* You peed in your underwear; you
                       should go to the restroom.

VAL   *[Sign]* I can't go; I have to take the test.

HUMPHREY   *[Sign]* Traci, Val, why are you talking?

TRACI   *(Points to Val's pats) [Sign]* Val's pants are wet.
                       He needs to go to the restroom.

HUMPHREY   *[Sign]* Val, why didn't you go to restroom?

VAL   *[Sign]* I had to take the test.

HUMPHREY   *[Sign]* Well, I want you to stay after class. I
                       need to talk to you about your pants. Please
                       continue to take the test.

VAL   *(Fusses with Traci) [Sign]* Okay. Thanks, Traci.

Val is forced to stay in the classroom after class. Humphrey talks to him about getting his pants wet.

HUMPHREY	*[Sign]* Val, I know why your pants got wet. If you need to use the restroom, you should go.
VAL	*[Sign]* I am so sorry, I can't help it.
HUMPHREY	*[Sign]* Please be a big boy, like Alan. When you feel like you need to, you have to go to the restroom.
VAL	*[Sign]* Okay, my bed was wet too.
HUMPHREY	*[Sign]* You didn't wake up to pee?
VAL	*[Sign]* No, I had to sleep.
HUMPHREY	*[Sign]* Please listen to me, if you don't want everyone to think you are a baby, you have to use the restroom.
VAL	*[Sign]* Okay, I will try my best.
HUMPHREY	*[Sign]* I think you need to change your pants before anyone else sees it. Please be careful.
VAL	*[Sign]* Do you love me even if my pants are wet?
HUMPHREY	*[Sign]* Of course, I love you no matter what. I don't want anyone to make fun of you for having wet pants.
VAL	*[Sign]* Okay, Humphrey. I will go to the restroom when I feel the need.
HUMPHREY	*[Sign]* Good boy. It is time to go to the dorm.

It is Sunday evening of December, 1976, Cole sees Val walking to the classroom and follows him. Cole sees Humphrey there.

COLE	*[Voice]* Hello Humphrey, I am so sorry if Val is bothering you. I better take him to the dorm.
HUMPHREY	*[Voice]* No, I invited him to come here to help me decorate the Christmas tree for our class.
COLE	*[Voice and sign]* Aww, sweet. Val, you can stay here.
VAL	*[Sign]* Thanks, Cole.
COLE	*[Voice]* I have to get something to eat for him.
HUMPHEY	*(Shows the bag to Cole) [Voice]* I have pimento cheese sandwiches and chocolate milk. He will eat them when we are done with the decorations.
COLE	*[Voice]* Sure, no problem. Have fun!
VAL	*[Sign]* Cole, you were right about Humphrey. She is sweet and kind, like you are.
COLE	*(Laughs) [Sign]* Great! Can you let me see the Christmas tree when it is decorated?
VAL	*[Sign]* Humphrey, is it okay with you?
HUMPHREY	*[Sign]* Sure, you can get her when it is done.

Cole leaves and Val helps Humphrey decorate the Christmas tree. Val laughs as they put the lights on, and he tells Humphrey he loves decorating the Christmas tree. Val eats the pimento cheese sandwiches and gets Cole to come see the Christmas tree. Cole is surprised and says it is beautiful. Val hugs Humphrey.

Scene Ten: Snow Day

It is snowing, the students look at the snow through the windows and get excited. Humphrey wonders where Val is.

Humphrey's Classroom

HUMPHREY	*[Sign]* Wow! It is snowing. Are you all excited?
CINDY	*[Sign]* It is beautiful, I love snow. Can we play outside?
HUMPHREY	*[Sign]* Sure, but all of you need to wear hats and coats before going outside. Where is Val?
SIMMONS	*(Shows up, looking upset) [Voice]* I saw Val dancing outside. He refused to come in.
HUMPHREY	*[Voice]* Where is he?
SIMMONS	*[Voice]* He went to the infirmary, then he came back, but he stayed outside in the snow.
HUMPHREY	*[Voice]* I will go get him. He is crazy about the snow.
SIMMONS	*[Voice]* Okay, get him in here while I stay with the students.
HUMPHREY	*[Sign]* Kids, please stay with Miss Simmons.

Mrs. Humphrey goes to the hallway and finds Val outside Eagles Hall, across from Woodard Hall. Val dances and enjoys the snow, Humphrey enjoys watching him. Val keeps laughing and saying how much he loves snow. Humphrey is in tears, laughing.

SIMMONS	*(Shows up) [Voice]* Why are you letting him dance in the snow? It is very cold out here.

HUMPHREY   *[Voice]* Look at him, I've never see him so happy before.

SIMMONS   *[Voice]* I see he is very happy, but he needs to go back to class.

HUMPHREY   *[Voice]* Oh, I thought you wanted him in your office.

SIMMONS   *(Sighs and leaves) [Voice]* I don't want to ruin his happy day. Get him to go to class.

HUMPHREY   *[Voice]* Thanks so much, I will get him.

HUMPHREY   *(Walks to Val and tags him) [Sign]* Val, I know you enjoy dancing in the snow, but it is very cold here and time to go to class.

VAL   *[Sign]* Okay, can we make snow cream? Our class will love it!

HUMPHREY   *[Sign]* Oh, have you eaten snow cream before?

VAL   *[Sign]* Yes, it tastes like ice cream. Yummy!

HUMPHREY   *[Sign]* Okay, we will make it as soon as we go back to class.

VAL   *[Sign]* Good, can we get a bowl for the snow?

HUMPHREY   *[Sign]* Okay, let's get it. We will love eating snow cream.

Back in the classroom, Val and Mrs. Humphrey make snow cream as the other students watch them.

CINDY   *[Sign]* I've never seen him so happy before. He must love snow cream!

TRACI	*[Sign]* I enjoy seeing him happy.
HUMPHREY	*[Sign]* Yes, he loves snow. He wants to help us make snow cream.
JUNIOR	*[Sign]* What is snow cream? I never tasted it before.
VAL	*[Sign]* It will taste like ice cream.
JUNIOR	*[Sign]* It looks look vanilla ice cream, I guess I will taste it.
VAL	*[Sign]* Everyone, eat snow cream. Enjoy it!
TRACI	*[Sign]* You are right, it is very good, like ice cream.
CAROLINA	*[Sign]* I love it. Thanks so much Humphrey.
HUMPHREY	*[Sign]* Great, you can thank Val because it was his idea to make snow cream for all of you.
THE STUDENTS	*[Sign]* Thanks so much Val! We love snow cream! *(Tap and hug Val)*
VAL	*[Sign]* You're welcome. It made today the best!
HUMPHREY	*[Sign]* It can be one of your best days at the school!
SIMMONS	*(Shows up and looks at the snow cream) [Voice]* Hello, how is the snow cream going?
HUMPHREY	*[Voice]* Great! They love eating it.
SIMMONS	*[Voice]* That's wonderful! I would like to taste snow cream.

VAL   *[Sign]* Here is some for you. Hope you are
               not mad at me anymore.

SIMMONS   *[Sign]* Val, thanks so much; I am not mad
               anymore. The snow cream made me happy.

*It is March 1977, the students are flying their kites at the Eagles Hall
playground. Val runs and flies his kite as Humphrey looks on. Val keeps
saying he can do it himself and Humphrey laughs.*

*In the spring, Humphrey and the students find out Val didn't come to school
on Sunday. On Monday, Val and his mother show up with an Easter tree.
The students are very pleased to see their names on the tree.*

*In the classroom, Humphrey brings chicken eggs and keeps them warm. Val
points out that an egg hatched. When the chicks grow up, they are sad to see
them go to the farm.*

Scene Eleven: Substitute Teacher

Val goes to Simmons' office and tags her.

SIMMONS   *[Sign]* Val, what are you doing? I am on the
               phone.

VAL   *[Sign]* Something is wrong with Humphrey.

SIMMONS   *[Sign]* Really? What's wrong?

VAL   *[Sign]* She fainted. She doesn't feel well; please
               come with me.

SIMMONS   *[Sign]* Okay, I am coming with you.

*Humphrey is forced to go home and rest. Her husband and sons take care of
her. She has the flu. She gets a call from Miss Simmons.*

HUMPHREY   *[Voice]* Hello, this is the Humphrey residence.
               Who is it?

SIMMONS   *[Voice]* Hello, it is me. How do you feel?

HUMPHREY   *[Voice]* The doctor said I have the flu. I am so
                   sorry I am not able to teach the students
                   tomorrow.

SIMMONS   *[Voice]* It is alright, I think you better rest for
                   now. I got a substitute for tomorrow.

HUMPHREY   *[Voice]* Thanks, who?

SIMMONS   *[Voice]* Her name is Miss Ezzard, she is a
                   student teacher. I am sure she will do well;
                   she will graduate soon.

HUMPHREY   *[Voice]* That sounds good. How is Val doing?

SIMMONS   *[Voice]* He is alright. He keeps asking me
                   about you. He must be worried.

HUMPHREY   *[Voice]* I understand how he feels. Do me a
                   favor.

SIMMONS   *[Voice]* Sure, what is it?

HUMPHREY   *[Voice]* Tell him I want him to listen to what
                   Miss Ezzard teaches, like he listens to me.

SIMMONS   *[Voice]* Sure, I will do that. Please take care
                   and don't worry; everything will be alright.
                   Get well soon.

HUMPHREY   *[Voice]* Thanks Simmons, bye.

*Val and his classmates go to Humphrey's classroom and they realize
Humphrey is not there. Simmons walks in and asks them to sit at their
desks.*

Humphrey's Classroom

SIMMONS   *[Sign]* Good morning kids, Mrs. Humphrey is

	unable to teach you today. She has the flu.
THE STUDENTS	*[Sign]* We are sorry.
SIMMONS	*[Sign]* She needs rest for now. I have someone to take her place to teach you. *(Miss Ezzard shows up)* Here is Miss Ezzard, she is a student teacher. Tell her hello.
THE STUDENTS	*[Sign]* Hello, Miss Ezzard.
EZZARD	*[Sign]* Hello, I am very pleased to teach you. I know how much you miss Mrs. Humphrey, but she wants me to teach you for a while.
SIMMONS	*[Sign]* Please be nice to her and have a good day.
EZZARD	*[Voice]* Wait, Miss Simmons.
SIMMONS	*[Voice]* Yes, what is it?
EZZARD	*[Voice]* Is the boy with the hole in his neck named Val Melvin? You told me about him earlier.
SIMMONS	*[Voice to Ezzard and sign to Val]* Yes, he is. Thanks for reminding me. *(Turns to Val)* Val, Mrs. Humphrey wants you to listen to what Mrs. Ezzard teaches. Okay?
VAL	*[Sign]* Okay, I will.
SIMMONS	*[Sign to Val and voice to Miss Ezzard]* Good boy. Miss Ezzard, please call me if you have any problems, good luck to you. *(She leaves)*
EZZARD	*[Sign]* Are you ready to learn spelling?
CAROLINA	*[Sign]* I guess so.

EZZARD   *[Sign]* Junior, what about you?

JUNIOR   *[Sign]* Spelling is fun, but I like the true and
                false quizzes more.

EZZARD   *[Sign]* Hello Val, Simmons told me about you.

VAL   *[Sign]* What did she tell you about me?

EZZARD   *[Sign]* She told me about your trach and your
                recessed jaws, and that you only eat soft
                foods. I hope you accept me as your teacher.

VAL   *(Feels uncomfortable)* *[Sign]* Did she replace
                Humphrey with you?

EZZARD   *[Sign]* Yes, but it is just temporary. She will
                come back when she gets well.

VAL   *[Sign]* Well, good luck teaching.

EZZARD   *[Sign]* Aww, thanks. I am going to teach all of
                you something new.

*Miss Ezzard teaches the students about nouns, verbs, and adjectives. They
listen to what she says, but Val doesn't pay attention to her.*

VAL   *[Sign]* Traci, Miss Ezzard is boring.

TRACI   *[Sign]* Please be nice to her.

VAL   *[Sign]* She is different form Humphrey. She is
                not good.

TRACI   *[Sign]* Take it easy, don't say anything. She
                will get upset.

VAL   *[Sign]* Why don't we get rid of her?

TRACI   *[Sign]* Val stop!

EZZARD	*[Sign]* Traci and Val, why do you keep talking while I teach you? What are you talking about?
VAL	*[Sign]* Nothing.
TRACI	*[Sign]* Nothing.
EZZARD	*[Sign]* Well, I want you two to stay with me during recess.
TRACI	*[Sign]* That's not fair, Val did it first.
VAL	*[Sign]* Please don't tell Humphrey.
EZZARD	*[Sign]* I am so sorry, but it is too late. Please pay attention to me.
TRACI	*(Turns to Val) [Sign]* It is your fault. I am mad at you!

Miss Ezzard asks the students to go to recess in the gym, but Traci and Val stay in the classroom. Traci complains that Val started talking first. Miss Ezzard decides to let her go.

EZZARD	*[Sign]* Traci, you may go to recess with them now.
TRACI	*[Sign]* Thanks so much. Val, you are in trouble.
VAL	*[Sign]* Why do I have to stay with you?
EZZARD	*[Sign]* I am disappointed in you. Why didn't you pay attention to me?
VAL	*[Sign]* You are different from Mrs. Humphrey, I prefer her.
EZZARD	*[Sign]* What about me?

VAL	*[Sign]* I like you, but you are boring.
EZZARD	*[Sign]* Got it, go to Simmons' office now!
VAL	*[Sign]* Did I do something wrong? I like you.
EZZARD	*[Sign]* You said I am boring; you hurt my feelings. You are going to Simmons' office.

Miss Ezzard gets mad and grabs Val's arm. She takes him to Simmons' office and he is punished for not paying attention to Miss Ezzard. Simmons puts him in the corner and makes Val eat lunch in her office.

At the Humphrey residence, Humphrey is still on bed rest. CW is off from work and taking care of her. CW finds her disappointed after a call from Miss Simmons about Val.

CW	*[Voice]* Mary Sue, how are you feeling, now?
HUMPHREY	*[Voice]* I am a little better, but I am very disappointed in Val. Something happened at school.
CW	*[Voice]* What happened?
HUMPHREY	*[Voice]* Val behaved badly today, and he didn't obey Miss Ezzard. I need to talk to him about his behavior.
CW	*[Voice]* But you are sick.
HUMPHREY	*[Voice]* I know, I will stay here. I am going to call Cole to bring Val here, so I can talk to him.
CW	*[Voice]* I understand, but you don't want him to catch the flu. How can you talk to him?
HUMPHREY	*[Voice]* Don't worry, I will ask him not to get close to me.

CW	*[Voice]* When do you want Cole and Val to come here?
HUMPHREY	*[Voice]* This afternoon. I am going to call Cole now.

Cole takes Val to the Humphrey residence and CW lets them come in. Val is very happy to see him and hugs him. CW tells him that Humphrey is in bed and wants to talk to him; Cole sits on the couch to wait for him.

VAL	*[Sign]* Hey Humphrey, I am very happy to see you. How do you feel?
HUMPHREY	*[Sign]* I am doing okay. Please don't hug me because I don't want you to get sick.
VAL	*[Sign]* Okay, Cole told me that you need to talk to me about something important.
HUMPHREY	*[Sign]* That's right. Please sit down on the chair.
VAL	*(Sits down) [Sign]* Why are you mad?
HUMPHREY	*[Sign]* I am disappointed that you treated Miss Ezzard badly. She worked hard to teach you.
VAL	*[Sign]* But she is different from you, she is boring.
HUMPHREY	*[Sign]* That is not a nice thing to say. I want you to listen to what she teaches you. She is a very good teacher.
VAL	*[Sign]* Okay, what do you want me to do?
HUMPHREY	*[Sign]* Tell her you are sorry. You have to pay attention to her and be nice to her.
VAL	*[Sign]* Okay, I will do that, I am very sorry.

HUMPHREY	*[Sign]* Me too, it upset me. I cried.
VAL	*[Sign]* I am so sorry. I will be nice to her. Do you love me?
HUMPHREY	*[Sign]* I still love you, but I am disappointed in you. I will be very happy if you obey Miss Ezzard.
VAL	*[Sign]* Okay, I will fix something for her.
HUMPHREY	*[Sign]* What?
VAL	*[Sign]* I will draw a picture, to make her happy.
HUMPHREY	*[Sign]* That sounds good. I remember that you drew some pictures for me.
VAL	*[Sign]* Yes, I am glad you liked them. Do you need rest?
HUMPHREY	*[Sign]* Yes, I need to get better. I will see you later, and I love you.
VAL	*[Sign]* Okay, I love you too.
HUMPHREY	*[Sign]* Val?
VAL	*[Sign]* Yes?
HUMPHREY	*[Sign]* Please listen to Miss Ezzard and be nice to her.
VAL	*[Sign]* Okay, I will do that. Thanks.

The next morning, the students sit at the class table. Val feels bad about yesterday and looks at, then taps, Traci.

VAL	*[Sign]* Good morning Traci, I need to talk to you.

TRACI	*[Sign]* Please leave me alone, I don't want to talk to you again. You behaved badly yesterday.
VAL	*[Sign]* I am so sorry about yesterday. I will tell Miss Ezzard that I am sorry. I have something for her.
TRACI	*[Sign]* Really, what made you change your mind?
VAL	*[Sign]* Humphrey.
TRACI	*[Sign]* You visited her? She is sick.
VAL	*[Sign]* Yes, Cole took me to see her. She wanted to talk to me. She is not happy about yesterday.
TRACI	*[Sign]* Oh, I hope you learned your lesson. What did you make?
VAL	*[Sign]* This is a picture I drew for Miss Ezzard. I want her to forgive me for what happened.
TRACI	*[Sign]* Aww, sweet. Here she comes.
EZZARD	*(Shows up) [Sign]* Good morning kids, I am so sorry I am late.
VAL	*(Runs to her and hugs her) [Sign]* Good morning, Miss Ezzard. Here is a picture I made for you, I hope you like it.
EZZARD	*[Sign]* Aww sweet. Thanks so much.
STEPHEN	*[Sign]* Why does he keep hugging her?
JUNIOR	*[Sign]* He wants to show how sorry he is.

VAL   *[Sign]* Miss Ezzard, I need to tell you
                           something important. I am very sorry about
                           yesterday. I will listen to what you say and I
                           will be nice to you.

EZZARD   *[Sign]* How very sweet of you; I appreciate
                           that. Val, please take a seat.

VAL   *[Sign]* Okay. *(Takes seat)* I am ready for your
                           lesson.

EZZARD   *[Sign]* Good boy, I have a question for you.

VAL   *[Sign]* Sure, ask me anything.

EZZARD   *[Sign]* Why did you change your mind about
                           me?

VAL   *[Sign]* I visited Humphrey and I had a
                           discussion with her. She asked me to listen
                           to you.

EZZARD   *[Sign]* That sounds great! I am glad you
                           learned your lesson. Okay, I am ready to
                           teach you all something new.

VAL   *(Raises his hand)* *[Sign]* Ezzard?

EZZARD   *[Sign]* Yes, Val?

VAL   *[Sign]* Why don't we make a get well card for
                           Humphrey? I am sure she will like it.

EZZARD   *[Sign]* That sounds like a good idea. Kids, do
                           you want to do that for Humphrey?

The students nod their heads.

EZZARD   *[Sign]* Val, we will do that if you pay
                           attention to me. We will make the card after
                           lunch. Okay?

VAL	*[Sign]* Deal!
EZZARD	*(Laughs) [Sign]* Good! Thanks, I am going to teach you now.

After lunch, the students make a get well card for Humphrey as Miss Ezzard watches them. Miss Ezzard brings the card and visits Humphrey.

HUMPHREY	*(Opens the door) [Voice]* Hello, Miss Ezzard, you can come in.
EZZARD	*[Voice]* Hello, Humphrey. I am so sorry you are sick. Your students asked me to bring this card to you; I hope you enjoy it.
HUMPHREY	*[Voice]* Aww, thanks so much. I feel a little better. I am looking forward getting back to my students. They are like my children.
EZZARD	*(Laughs) [Voice]* I know how you feel. I am sure they are looking forward to having you back, especially Val. He asked me about you.
HUMPHREY	*[Voice]* That's great. How is he doing? Has Val been good for you?
EZZARD	*[Voice]* Yes, he is a very sweet boy. He told me he visited you, and you made him listen to what I say.
HUMPHREY	*[Voice]* Yes, I talked to him. I made him do that for me. I am glad that he was a good boy. What did Val do today?
EZZARD	*[Voice]* He did math work, he is very good at math. I know you helped him with it.
HUMPHREY	*[Voice]* Yes, I had a hard time with him when school started. He was lazy, but his grades and progress have improved. I work hard to

help him.

EZZARD   *[Voice]* That's great. I am glad you get along
                  well. Please let me know when you are ready
                  to come back to school.

HUMPHREY   *[Voice]* Okay, I will let you know. Thanks so
                  much for subbing for me. I appreciate it.

EZZARD   *[Voice]* Thanks, again. Have a good evening.

*The next morning, Val and his classmates go to the classroom and look at
the blackboard. It say: "Guess who is back." The students look puzzled
until Humphrey shows up.*

HUMPHREY   *[Sign]* Good morning, students. I am back
                  and I feel better now. Thanks so much for
                  the card.

The students run to her and hug her. She laughs as Val hugs her.

VAL   *[Sign]* We are very happy to have you again.
                  Where is Miss Ezzard? I would like to see
                  her again.

HUMPHREY   *[Sign]* She is back in college for her final
                  exams. Hopefully we will see her again. I am
                  proud of you for paying attention to her.

VAL   *[Sign]* Aww, I miss her. I hope she is alright.

HUMPHREY   *[Sign]* Please sit down. It is time for class to
                  start.

Scene Twelve: Hide and Seek

The next day, the students play hide and seek at the Eagles Hall playground. Kathy closes her eyes and counts to 20 while the kids run and hide. Kathy opens her eyes and looks for her classmates. She finds some of them.

The Eagles Hall Playground

KATHY *(Touches Traci) [Sign]* Traci! I found you!

TRACI *[Sign]* Aw, nuts. I thought I hid well.

KATHY *(Points to Cindy) [Sign]* Cindy, I got you.

CINDY *[Sign]* Aw, nuts. Hope you find the others.

Kathy finds the other students. They meet at the wall where Kathy closed her eyes and counted.

KATHY *[Sign]* This was fun. Want to play more?

JUNIOR *[Sign]* But Val is missing, we have to find him.

KATHY *[Sign]* He is very good at hiding.

JUNIOR *[Sign]* Okay, we are going to find him before we go back to the classroom. I hope he is alright.

The kids look for Val, and Carolina finds his shoe at the base of a tree. She looks up and sees Val sitting in the tree.

HUMPHREY *[Sign]* Come on, kids, recess is over. It is time to go back to class now.

The students don't say anything.

HUMPHREY *(Looks for Val) [Sign]* Where is Val? Have you seen him?

CAROLINA   *(Holds one of Val's shoes)* *[Sign]* I just found
                    one of his shoes.

HUMPHREY   *[Sign]* Kids, please don't tell me Val is lost.

TRACI   *[Sign]* No, he is not lost. I don't want you to
                    get mad at him. We know where he is.

HUMPHREY   *[Sign]* Tell me where he is. Please.

The students look at each other and turn to Mrs. Humphrey. They clear their throats.

JUNIOR   *[Sign]* Okay, please come with us and we will
                    show you.

Humphrey follows her students to the tree and Junior points to Val. Humphrey looks up at Val and screams.

HUMPHREY   *[Sign]* Val! How did you get there?

VAL   *[Sign]* I climbed up. It was easy.

HUMPHREY   *(Gets mad)* *[Sign]* You scared me! Please get
                    down.

VAL   *[Sign]* Okay, *(Gets down)* I am so sorry.

HUMPHREY   *[Sign]* Kids, go back to the classroom. *(Turns
                    to Val)* I want you to stay with me after class
                    and we will have a talk.

VAL   *[Sign]* Am I bad?

HUMPHREY   *(Holds Val's hand)* *[Sign]* Yes, you are a bad
                    boy. Climbing the tree is dangerous for you.
                    Let's go back to the classroom.

Humphrey pulls Val's arm and they go to the classroom. She puts Val in the corner. After class, the students leave and go to the dorm. Humphrey walks to Val and hugs him.

HUMPHREY	*[Sign]* Your punishment is over, it is time to go to the dorm.
VAL	*[Sign]* Okay, why are you mad at me?
HUMPHREY	*[Sign]* I don't want you to climb the tree because it is dangerous. You need to be careful and not get hurt.
VAL	*[Sign]* Okay, I understand. Alan taught me how.
HUMPHREY	*[Sign]* Really? Do your parents know he taught you how to climb? How long have you been climbing?
VAL	*[Sign]* Since last Saturday. I watched him climb, that's all.
HUMPHREY	*[Sign]* Well, he made a mistake. Your brother is older and bigger than you. You should not climb trees.
VAL	*[Sign]* If you don't want me to climb again, I won't.
HUMPHREY	*[Sign]* Good boy. It is time to go the dorm. See you tomorrow, I am not mad anymore.
VAL	*(Hugs Humphrey) [Sign]* Thanks so much Humphrey. See you tomorrow.

Humphrey walks in the hallway and stops to see Cole in her office.

COLE	*[Voice]* Hello Humphrey, I heard about what happened. I hope Val is alright.
HUMPHREY	*[Voice]* Yes, he is fine. It scared me when I saw him up in that tree, I don't want him to climb again.

COLE   *[Voice]* I know what you mean. His parents wouldn't want him to climb; why did he do it?

HUMPHREY   *[Voice]* He watched Alan climb a tree.

COLE   *[Voice]* Got it, we need to call his parents and let them know what happened today.

HUMPHREY   *[Voice]* No way, I don't want to scare them. Alan is the only family member I haven't meet. I wonder when we will get to meet him.

COLE   *[Voice]* You will meet him soon.

HUMPHREY   *[Voice]* Really, when?

COLE   *[Voice]* Wait and see.

HUMPHREY   *[Voice]* Okay, thanks; have a good evening.

Scene Thirteen: Val's Brother Visits

On Friday afternoon, Val and the students eat spaghetti and meat sauce. Val cuts it as Humphrey looks on. She tells Val she is proud of him for cutting his food before he eats. Humphrey sees Cole, who is waving and she tells the students she will be back.

COLE   *[Voice]* We have a visitor, it is Alan. Mrs. Melvin went to Wilson to meet someone and Alan wanted to have lunch with his little brother.

HUMPHREY   *[Voice]* Sure, no problem. *(Turns to Alan)* Hi, Alan. I am very pleased to meet you. Val told me lots about you.

ALAN   *[Voice]* Hello Mrs. Humphrey. Where is Val?

I want to have lunch with him.

HUMPHREY   *[Voice]* Sure, come with me. *(Turns to Cole)*
                  Thanks, Cole.

*Humphrey takes Alan to the lunchroom and goes to the table. Val is
surprised to see his brother and hugs him.*

The Eagles Hall Lunchroom

VAL   *[Sign]* Alan, are you hungry?

ALAN   *[Sign to Val and voice to Humphrey]* Yes, I am.
                  (Turns to Humphrey) Can I sit next to him?
                  Thanks!

HUMPHREY   *[Voice to Alan and sign to Val]* Yes, you can.
                  Let me get some food for you. *(Turns to Val)*
                  Please introduce your classmates to Alan.

VAL   *(Turns to his classmates)* *[Sign]* This is my
                  brother Alan. He is here to have lunch with
                  us.

TRACI   *[Sign]* Yes, he can. He seems very nice.

HUMPHREY   *[Voice]* Alan, here is your chair, sit down.

ALAN   *[Voice]* Thanks Humphrey, where is my
                  food?

HUMPHREY   *[Voice]* It will be here soon. Please be
                  patient.

SIMMONS   *[Voice]* Hello Humphrey, who is the visitor?

HUMPHREY   *[Voice]* This is Alan, Val's brother. He is here
                  to have lunch with us while Mrs. Melvin is in
                  Wilson meeting someone. She will be here
                  around three.

VAL	*[Sign]* Alan, this is Miss Simmons. She is our principal.
ALAN	*[Voice]* Hello Simmons, nice to meet you.
SIMMONS	*[Voice]* Thanks, you too. Enjoy your lunch.
VAL	*[Sign]* Mrs. Humphrey, thanks so much for letting Alan stay with us for lunch. I am very happy.
HUMPHREY	*[Sign]* Welcome, anytime. I wanted to meet him. He can go to the infirmary with you after lunch, if he wants.
VAL	*[Sign]* Sure, thanks.

Alan's food arrives. They eat spaghetti and meat sauce. After, Alan and Val go to the infirmary and then to the classroom. The students sit at the class table while Alan sits in Val's chair. The students are doing math.

Humphrey's Classroom

VAL	*[Sign]* Humphrey, Alan is lonely.
HUMPHREY	*[Sign]* Don't worry, I will keep him company while you do math work.
VAL	*[Sign]* Okay.
HUMPHREY	*(Walks to Alan) [Voice]* Hello, Alan. Val doesn't want to see you lonely so I will keep you company. How are you doing?
ALAN	*[Voice]* Doing fine, thanks. This school is different from mine, but it looks very nice.
HUMPHREY	*[Voice]* Right, it is very different. How do you feel when Val is not around?
ALAN	*[Voice]* It's strange, I feel like I am an only

child. I sleep in his bed sometimes.

HUMPHREY   *[Voice]* I know how you feel, you miss him. Did you two go to the infirmary after lunch?

ALAN   *[Voice]* Yes, we did. Val pointed out a tree to me, is it the one he climbed?

HUMPHREY   *[Voice]* Yes, he scared me when I saw him in the tree. I didn't want him to fall down, but he climbed down and is fine now.

ALAN   *[Voice]* Oh no, it is my fault. I forgot my parents didn't want him to climb trees. It is dangerous.

HUMPHREY   *[Voice]* Please don't feel bad. You can climb, but you have to tell him that it is not good for him.

ALAN   *[Voice]* I understand. Please don't tell my parents.

HUMPHREY   *[Voice]* Wait a minute, they don't know you climb?

ALAN   *[Voice]* No, I just learned to climb. It is just a Scout thing. I don't want to upset them.

HUMPHREY   *[Voice]* You have to tell your parents that you climb, but you don't have to tell them about Val. We will keep our secret.

ALAN   *[Voice]* Thanks, I will. It looks like you care about Val. You teach him well. He has learned a lot; I am proud of him.

HUMPHREY   *[Voice]* I didn't give up on him until I helped him learn.

ALAN   *[Voice]* You are the best teacher Val has. Val

has friends here and they accept who he is.

HUMPHREY   *[Voice]* That's right. Were you worried about him?

ALAN   *[Voice]* Yes, I was very worried, but he is happy here, thanks to you.

HUMPHREY   *(Smiles)* *[Voice]* Yes, he is very happy. He enjoys learning.

VAL   *[Sign]* I am finished with math, it is easy for me.

HUMPHREY   *[Sign]* Thanks Val, can you show Alan some sign language books? He can borrow them so he can communicate with you.

VAL   *[Sign]* Okay, come with me Alan.

Val shows Alan the sign language books and asks if he wants to borrow some of them. He signs to him yes. Humphrey looks at them and is very happy she was able to meet Alan.

Scene Fourteen: Good News about Val's Grades

One week later, the students are at the classroom and the lights go out because lightning hits a nearby pole. Val is scared and runs and hides under his desk.

HUMPHREY   *[Sign]* Val, you okay?

VAL   *[Sign]* I am scared of lightening, I can feel it.

HUMPHREY   *[Sign]* You can feel it?

VAL   *[Sign]* Yes, I can feel it. It hit me.

HUMPHREY   *[Sign]* Please take it easy. It won't hurt you.

VAL   *[Sign]* Okay.

HUMPHREY   *[Sign]* Come on, stay with me. Kids, I know all of you are scared of the lighting.

TRACI   *[Sign]* Does it kill people?

HUMPHREY   *[Sign]* I am afraid so, but stay inside and you will be safe.

VAL   *[Sign]* What if I need to go to the infirmary?

HUMPHREY   *[Sign]* You don't have to go until the weather is back to normal. Then you can go there.

VAL   *[Sign]* I feel safe with you.

HUMPHREY   *(Holds Val's hand)* *[Sign]* Dear, I am here with you.

One week later, Miss Simmons and Humphrey have a meeting with Val's parents in her office. They discuss his grades and progress. Simmons asks Humphrey to get Val from the TV room.

HUMPHREY   *[Sign]* You can come with me to see your parents, the meeting is over.

VAL   *[Sign]* Did I do something wrong?

HUMPHREY   *[Sign]* No, you did nothing wrong. We just discussed your grades, that's all.

VAL   *[Sign]* Are my grades good?

HUMPHREY   *(Holds Val's hand)* *[Sign]* Wait and see. Come with me.

Humphrey escorts Val to Simmons' office. His parents are excited and hug Val.

VAL   *[Sign]* Mama, Papa, why are you so excited?

FALLON   *(Turns to Simmons) [Voice]* Simmons, why don't you tell him?

SIMMONS   *[Sign]* Okay, Mr. Melvin. *(Turns to Val)* I have good news for your parents. I told them you did an excellent job with your grades, you have made many improvements. Everything has changed because of Humphrey.

VAL   *[Sign]* I know, she helps me learn.

BETTY   *[Sign to Val and voice to Humphrey]* We don't know what to say, but thanks so much Humphrey. You did a wonderful job.

HUMPHREY   *[Voice]* Welcome anytime, it is my job to teach him.

BETTY   *[Sign]* Val, what do you say to Humphrey?

VAL   *[Sign]* Thanks, Humphrey. I love you.

HUMPHREY   *[Sign to Val and voice to Betty]* Aww, I love you too. *(Turns to Betty)* Is it okay if he tells me he loves me?

BETTY   *(Laughs) [Voice]* I'm not jealous. He knows you care about him because you worked hard to help him.

FALLON   *[Voice]* It is fine with us, I am glad you two love each other.

VAL   *[Sign]* I love her because she is the best teacher I have.

BETTY   *[Sign]* That's right, she is.

FALLON   *[Sign]* It is time to go, we will go out to eat to celebrate.

FALLON   *[Voice]* Okay, I will pay for lunch, then we
                    will let you go.

CW   *[Voice]* Excuse me, you don't have to pay.

FALLON   *[Voice]* That's what my wife and I want to do
                    because your wife worked so hard to help
                    Val learn.

CW   *[Voice]* I hate to object but…

HUMPHREY   *(Takes her husband aside) [Voice]* Please accept,
                    we will buy them lunch next time.

FALLON   *[Voice]* Your wife is right. A deal is a deal!

CW   *(Laughs) [Voice]* I am so sorry. I don't like
                    anyone treating us to lunch, but I know how
                    much you and your wife appreciate what
                    Mary Sue did for your son. Thanks so much.

VAL   *[Sign]* I am not finished; I will eat chocolate
                    pie.

HUMPHREY   *(Teases) [Sign]* You are going to get fat.
                    Thomas and Blaine will be home soon and
                    waiting for us. We enjoyed having lunch
                    with you.

VAL   *[Sign]* Okay, tell them I said hello. See you
                    on Monday, I love you.

HUMPHREY   *(Hugs Val) [Sign]* Okay, I will do that. I love
                    you too, have a great weekend.

BETTY   *(Hugs Humphrey) [Voice]* Thanks so much for
                    everything. See you later.

FALLON   *(Shakes CW's hand) [Voice]* Pleased to meet
                    you, I hope to see you again.

CW   *[Voice]* We will, and thanks again. Be careful
                            driving home.

They leave as Val's parents look at him eating his chocolate pie.

BETTY   *[Sign]* You don't have to hurry. Please take
                            your time.

VAL   *[Sign]* But Alan is waiting for us.

BETTY   *[Sign]* Don't worry, he is with his friend.
                            Finish your dessert.

Scene Fifteen: The Last Day of Class

*Miss Bass asks Val to go to Cole's office. Val wears his pajamas and robe
and finds Cole at her desk. Mrs. Cole gets some cake and milk for Val.*

Cole's Office

VAL   *[Sign]* Hello Cole, Miss Bass told me you
                            wanted to see me. Did I do something
                            wrong?

COLE   *(Laughs)* *[Sign]* No, you are a very good boy.
                            I wanted to invite you to come to my office
                            to eat cake with me for the last night at the
                            dorm before the summer.

VAL   *[Sign]* Aww sweet. Thanks, *(Eats cake)* it is
                            very good, what kind is it?

COLE   *[Sign]* Pound cake. I want you to eat it.

VAL   *[Sign]* You are very sweet. I have a reason
                            why I love you so much.

COLE   *[Sign]* Really, what is it?

VAL   *[Sign]* You don't spank me. I saw you spank some kids but not me. You don't want to spank me?

COLE   *(Clears her throat)* *[Sign]* I don't want to spank you because your parents are very kind and sweet to me.

VAL   *[Sign]* You put me in the corner instead.

COLE   *(Cries)* *[Sign]* That's right. *(Sniff)* I can't believe the school year is over.

VAL   *[Sign]* You okay? Why are you crying?

COLE   *[Sign]* Oh Val, I am going to miss you this summer.

VAL   *[Sign]* Me too, I will think about you. Do you live here?

COLE   *[Sign]* No, I live in Hookerton.

VAL   *[Sign]* Then why did you sleep in your room?

COLE   *[Sign]* Oh, I stay here five days and I go home for the weekend; I am going to stay in Hookerton for the summer.

VAL   *[Sign]* I bet you are happy that you are going home. I can't wait to be with my family for the summer.

COLE   *[Sign]* I know you are very excited. Are you going to miss Mrs. Humphrey too?

VAL   *[Sign]* Yes, so much. She looked quiet today, I think she is excited about summer.

COLE   *[Sign]* She is going to miss you.

VAL	*[Sign]* Yes, I love her. She is the best teacher I have had. I want to spend time with her this summer.
COLE	*[Sign]* Great! Why don't you ask her?
VAL	*[Sign]* Sure, I will. I have to go now, it is my bedtime.
COLE	*[Sign]* Alright, go to the dorm now. Good night.
VAL	*(Hugs Cole) [Sign]* Cole, I love you. Thanks so much for taking care of me. I will see you tomorrow, good night and thanks again for the cake.
COLE	*(In tears) [Sign]* Oh Val, I love you too. I'll never forget you are my little boy. See you tomorrow.

Val waves goodbye to Cole and walks in the hallway as Cole looks on in tears.

The next day, Humphrey and her students are having a farewell party. Val gives his classmates goodbye hugs before they leave. Val stays with Humphrey to wait for his mother to arrive.

Humphrey's Classroom

VAL	*[Sign]* I am excited to go home and stay with my family, but I will miss you.
HUMPHREY	*[Sign]* Me too, I want you to have fun this summer with them. I will think of you often.
BETTY	*(Shows up) [Sign]* Come on, Val.
VAL	*[Sign]* I will be back.
HUMPHREY	*[Sign]* Okay.

BETTY	*[Sign]* Val, please give these flowers to her and tell her how much you love her.
VAL	*[Sign]* Humphrey, this is for you.
HUMPHREY	*[Sign]* Oh my, I love it. It is beautiful; thanks so much.
VAL	*[Sign]* You are welcome. I have to tell you something.
HUMPHREY	*[Sign]* Sure, what is it?
VAL	*[Sign]* You changed my life. I know you worked hard and taught me well. You made me learn. I was very pleased to have a wonderful teacher like you. I will never forget you.
HUMPHREY	*[Sign]* Aww, how very sweet of you to say such kind words. I was very pleased to have you as my student. I will never forget you.

Val is in tears.

HUMPHREY	*[Sign]* You okay?
VAL	*[Sign]* I am crying a little. I was very nervous telling you about my feelings.
HUMPHREY	*[Sign]* It is okay, I feel same way.
VAL	*(In tears) [Sign]* I love you Mrs. Humphrey!
HUMPHREY	*[Sign]* Aww, oh Val, *(Tears and hugs Val)* I love you too!
BETTY	*[Sign to Val and voice to Humphrey]* Val, it is time to go home. Mrs. Humphrey, thanks so much for teaching him. My husband and I appreciate what you did for him, you are a

part of his life.

HUMPHREY	*[Voice]* Oh Mrs. Melvin, *(Hugs her)* I am glad Val has two wonderful parents like you and Mr. Melvin.
BETTY	*[Voice]* I know you will miss him, but you will see him again.
HUMPHREY	*[Voice]* Have fun this summer. See you in the fall.

Humphrey is in tears as Val and his mother leave. They go to Mrs. Cole's office to give her some flowers and Cole gives him a goodbye hug. They get ready to go home, but Humphrey stops them.

HUMPHREY	*[Voice]* Mrs. Melvin!
BETTY	*[Voice]* Yes, Humphrey?
HUMPHREY	*[Voice]* I have to ask you something, I hope you and your husband don't mind.
BETTY	*[Voice]* Sure, what is it?
HUMPHREY	*[Voice]* I wonder if Val could spend a few days with me and my family this summer. He is very special to me. Is it okay with you?
BETTY	*[Voice]* That's great, but we have a busy summer planned. We go to White Lake, and Val has an operation at Duke.
HUMPHREY	*(Looks disappointed)* *[Voice]* I understand.
BETTY	*[Voice]* Don't worry, Fallon and I will discuss Val's schedule, and maybe he can spend a few days with you. We will let you know.
HUMPHREY	*[Voice]* That's great, I'm looking forward to it.

BETTY	*[Voice]* You can tell Val about it now.
HUMPHREY	*[Turns to Val who is in the car) [Sign]* Val, I would like to ask you something special.
VAL	*[Sign]* Okay, what is it?
HUMPHREY	*[Sign]* Would you like to spend a few days with me and my family during the summer? It will be fun!
VAL	*[Sign]* Yes, I want to. I have to ask mama to see if it is okay with her.
BETTY	*[Sign]* Yes, we will talk about it later.
VAL	*(Gets out of the car and hugs Humphrey) [Sign]* Yay! I will see you again!
BETTY	*[Sign to Val and voice to Humphrey]* That's wonderful, get in the car. I will call you when we set a date.
HUMPHREY	*(Hugs her) [Voice]* Thanks so much Mrs. Melvin. We will keep in touch. Be careful driving home.
BETTY	*[Voice]* Thank you so much. See you soon.

Humphrey waves at Val and his mother as they leave.

Scene Sixteen: Humphrey's Summer Plan with Val

June 1977: Time with the Humphreys

Val and his father drive to Wilson to go to the Humphrey residence. He drops Val off there. Val is excited to be at the Humphrey house.

Humphrey Residence

VAL	*[Sign]* Humphrey! I am here to spend a few days with you. I know you are very happy to see me.
HUMPHREY	*(Hugs him) [Sign]* Welcome back to our house. We have some fun things planned.
FALLON	*[Sign]* Val, please behave for Mrs. Humphrey. Have fun and I love you.
VAL	*[Sign]* I will, I love you too, see you soon. *(Hugs his father)*
FALLON	*[Voice]* Please take care of my son. I hope you enjoy having him for a while, bye. *(He leaves)*
VAL	*[Sign]* Humphrey, what are we doing while I stay here?
HUMPHREY	*[Sign]* You will find out.

Val goes to the food store to help Humphrey pick up some food. Val finds pimento cheese and asks Humphrey if she can make sandwiches for lunch.

Val helps Humphrey make chocolate pudding. They laugh.

Val plays fetch with Humphrey's dog. He signs to the dog, but Humphrey tells Val that the dog can't read signs.

Val and the Humphrey family go to a baseball game, they enjoy watching the game. CW buys him a baseball cap.

Val and Humphrey go swimming, but Val is in the shallow pool because of his track. After, they stop to get a milkshake.

Thomas and Blaine help Val catch some fireflies. Val keeps signing "I wish Alan was here," but he is at summer camp.

Val and Humphrey go shopping where they run into some teachers from school. He finds Miss Simmons in a beauty shop.

Val enjoys seeing Humphrey's tomato garden and asks her if he can pick some tomatoes for his mother and Humphrey says okay. Val tell her they are her favorite vegetables and Humphrey laughs.

The living room at the Humphrey Residence.

Val walks to the living room and finds Humphrey sitting on the couch. Humphrey is quiet and sad.

VAL	*[Sign]* Humphrey, you okay? You look sad.
HUMPHREY	*[Sign]* I am sad that today is your last day with me. Your Mama and Papa are on their way to pick you up.
VAL	*[Sign]* Aww, do you want me to stay longer?
HUMPHREY	*[Sign]* I wish, but you need to go home because you have to go to the hospital for your surgery.
VAL	*[Sign]* I don't like the hospital. Why do they want me to have an operation again?
HUMPHREY	*[Sign]* They want you to look good. The doctor can do his best for you. Please be strong for me.
VAL	*[Sign]* Yes. Will you and CW come to the hospital to see me? Please?
HUMPHREY	*[Sign]* Yes, I will talk to your parents about it. Please sit on my lap.

VAL	*[Sign]* Me? Why?
HUMPHREY	*[Sign]* You know how much I love you. I need to hold you before you leave.
VAL	*[Sign]* I know you are very sad to see me leave. *(Sits on her lap)* Feel better?
HUMPHREY	*[Sign]* Thank you. That's a good boy.
VAL	*[Sign]* I wish I could live with you because all of you are sweet and kind.
HUMPHREY	*[Sign]* I know, but you are lucky to have Mama, Papa, and Alan as your loving, caring family.
VAL	*[Sign]* Yes, you and your family are a second family to me. I love all of you.
HUMPHREY	*[Sign]* We love you too, my boy.
CW	*[Voice]* Mary Sue, Fallon and Betty are here.

Val's parents arrive at the Humphrey's home. They discuss all of the things they did while Val was there. Val's parents get ready to take him home.

BETTY	*[Sign]* Val, it is time to go home. Say goodbye to Humphrey and tell her thanks.
VAL	*[Sign]* She is very sad to see me leave.
BETTY	*[Voice]* Aww, Humphrey, I know how much you love him. You and your husband can come to the hospital to see Val if you want.
HUMPHREY	*[Voice]* Oh, Betty, thanks so much! *(Hugs her)* Please let me know when the best time is to visit him.
BETTY	*[Voice to Humphrey and sign to Val]* I will call you after the operation. I am glad that he had fun with all of you. Thanks so much for taking

care of our son. Come on Val.

VAL *[Sign]* May I have some time with Mrs. Humphrey?

BETTY *[Sign]* Why?

VAL *[Sign]* I want to give her a big hug of thanks for what she did for me.

BETTY *[Sign]* Sure, go ahead.

VAL *(Hugs Humphrey) [Sign]* Humphrey, I had a great time with all of you. Thanks so much for taking me places. I love you.

HUMPHREY *(Hugs Val) [Sign]* I love you too. I enjoyed having you. Please be strong for me.

BETTY *[Sign]* Come on, Val we need to go.

VAL *[Sign]* I can't.

BETTY *[Sign]* Why not?

VAL *[Sign]* She holds me tighter. She doesn't want me to leave.

FALLON *[Voice]* CW?

CW *[Voice]* Okay. *(Turns to Humphrey)* Mary Sue, please let Val go. They have to go now.

FALLON *[Voice]* I know you are worried about his operation. Please pray for him and be strong. I will let you know how Val is doing.

HUMPHREY *[Voice to Val's parents and sign to Val]* Okay, *(Turns to Val)* I will pray for you and think of you.

VAL   *[Sign]* Thanks so much, I love you, bye.

BETTY   *[Voice]* Thanks Mary Sue, I will contact you
                       next week.

HUMPHREY   *[Voice]* Thanks Betty. Please be safe driving.
                       Talk to you later, bye.

Val and his parents leave as Humphrey is in tears watching them.

CW   *(Comforts his wife)* *[Voice]* Dear, please take it
                       easy. We will go see him in the hospital next
                       week.

HUMPHREY   *[Voice]* You are right, I am looking forward to
                       that.

Duke Hospital Room

*Val has bandages on his head after his operation. He is lying on the bed, but
Betty wakes him up to take a bath.*

BETTY   *[Sign]* You need to take a bath. Your visitors
                       will be here soon.

VAL   *[Sign]* Who?

BETTY   *[Sign]* Mrs. Humphrey and her husband. They
                       want to see how you are doing.

VAL   *[Sign]* Wow! I can't wait to see them. I can't
                       take a bath because I have the IV.

BETTY   *[Sign]* Don't worry, the nurse will help you.

FALLON   *[Sign]* You have two visitors, Mrs. Humphrey
                       and her husband are here to see you.

VAL   *[Sign]* CW! Mrs. Humphrey! I am very happy
                       to see you. Come in!

HUMPHREY   *[Sign]* Me too, I am very happy that you are
                  alright. Here is a gift!

VAL   *(Hugs her) [Sign]* Thanks so much, I love the
                  puzzle book.

BETTY   *[Voice]* I am glad you are here. I know Val is
                  very happy to see you; I am pleased to have
                  you.

FALLON   *[Voice]* You okay?

BETTY   *[Voice]* I am doing alright.

HUMPHREY   *[Voice]* Your eyes are red, you look very tired.

BETTY   *[Voice]* I spent the night here. The nurse kept
                  waking us up when she checked on Val.

HUMPHREY   *[Voice]* Fallon?

FALLON   *[Voice]* Yes, Mary Sue?

HUMPHREY   *[Voice]* I think you better take her out
                  somewhere so she can relax. We will stay with
                  Val.

FALLON   *[Voice]* Good idea. Why don't we go now?

BETTY   *[Voice]* I can't leave Val.

FALLON   *[Voice]* Mary Sue said she and her husband will
                  stay with Val so we can go out.

HUMPHREY   *[Voice]* Please go to the hotel and take a nap.
                  We will stay with Val. Please trust me.

BETTY   *[Voice to Humphrey and sign to Val]* You are
                  right. Thanks so much Humphrey. *(Hugs
                  Humphrey)* Val, we have to go now; I need to
                  rest. Have a great time with Humphrey.

VAL	*(Kisses his mama) [Sign]* Okay, I love you.
BETTY	*[Sign to Val and voice to Humphrey]* I love you too, see you soon. *(Turns to Humphrey)* Please take care of him.
HUMPHREY	*[Voice]* Sure, we will. Get some rest.

Val's parents leave as Val looks on.

VAL	*[Sign]* Why do they have to go?
HUMPHREY	*[Sign]* Your parents need to go out, and your mother needs some sleep because she was up last night.
VAL	*[Sign]* You are right, but I am happy you two are here. I don't like to be alone.
HUMPHREY	*[Sign]* I understand. We are here with you.
THE DIETARY	*(Shows up with food for Val) [Voice as Humphrey signs to Val]* Here is your lunch, I hope you will enjoy it.
HUMPHREY	*(Opens the dish) [Sign]* It smells very good.
VAL	*(Pushes the food away) [Sign]* Phew! I don't like it.
HUMPHREY	*[Sign]* Oh, I thought you liked vegetables. Don't you love them?
VAL	*[Sign]* Yes, sometimes they are good, but not at the hospital. Hospital food is yucky. I don't like it.
HUMPHREY	*[Sign]* They are vegetables, they are good for you. Please try them.
VAL	*[Sign]* I don't like to fight with you. You taught me well.

HUMPHREY	*[Sign]* Good boy, please eat them. It will help you feel better.
VAL	*(Eats the hospital food) [Sign]* They are good. It is same as the lunchroom at school.
HUMPHREY	*[Sign]* Good boy! I am proud of you.
VAL	*(Eats his lunch) [Sign]* I am finished, they were good.
HUMPHREY	*[Sign]* Why don't you take a nap?
NURSE	*(Shows up) [Voice]* Hello, I hate to say this, but it is time for Val to walk around.
HUMPHREY	*[Sign]* She wants you to walk around.
VAL	*[Sign]* I want to stay in the bed.
HUMPHREY	*[Sign]* I think walking is important for you; you need to keep walking around if you want to go home.
VAL	*[Sign]* Home? I want to go home to see Alan.
HUMPHREY	*[Sign]* Yes, you will go home soon if you walk.
VAL	*[Sign]* What about the IV?
HUMPHREY	*[Sign]* I will hold the IV machine while you walk around.
VAL	*[Sign]* Okay, please get my slippers and a robe.
HUMPHREY	*[Sign]* Here they are. Let me help you get them on.
VAL	*(Laughs) [Sign]* You are like a second mother to me because you care about me.

HUMPHREY   *(Laughs) [Sign]* That's right. Ready to get up and walk?

VAL   *(Nods his head) [Sign]* Look at CW, he is sleeping.

HUMPHREY   *[Sign]* He must be tired from the trip. The traffic was heavy.

CW   *(Wakes up) [Voice]* Where are you going?

HUMPHREY   *[Voice and sign]* We are going for a walk. Val needs to walk around to get better so he can go home.

VAL   *[Sign]* You can take a nap if you want.

CW   *[Voice as Humphrey signs to Val]* Do you think I am lazy?

Val and Mrs. Humphrey look at each other and laugh.

CW   *[Voice as Humphrey signs to Val]* That's funny! I want to go with you. I want to make sure he is doing well.

HUMPHREY   *[Sign and voice]* You don't have to worry about him. I will take care of him.

VAL   *[Sign]* Humphrey, let him come with me. He loves me too.

CW   *[Voice]* That's right, I love him like another son. Let's go for a walk. Do we go outside?

HUMPHREY   *[Voice]* No, we just walk in the hallway. Is that okay?

CW   *[Voice]* Okay. Let's go.

Val and the Humphreys walk in the hallway as Humphrey holds the IV machine for him. Val greets the other patients by waving at them.

CW	*[Voice]* Look at him, he loves greeting the children.
HUMPHREY	*[Voice]* Yes, he is a fighter.
VAL	*[Sign]* I enjoy walking here. I feel strong.
HUMPHREY	*[Sign]* Great, I bet you are almost ready to go home.

Val walks into the kitchen as Humphrey looks on.

HUMPHREY	*[Sign]* Hey, where are you going? You have to ask someone first.
VAL	*[Sign]* Ask the nurse if I can have ice cream.
HUMPHREY	*[Sign]* Sure, but I thought you were full?
VAL	*[Sign]* It is for my dessert.
HUMPHREY	*(Laughs) [Sign]* Oh, Val you are spoiled.
NURSE	*[Voice]* May I help you?
HUMPHREY	*[Voice]* This patient wants some ice cream. I think he wants chocolate.
NURSE	*[Voice]* Sure. *(Gets ice cream from the freezer and gives it to Val)* Here it is, enjoy.
VAL	*[Sign]* Thanks, I need to go to my room, so I can eat my ice cream.
HUMPHREY	*[Sign]* Okay, let's go.

They go back to the hospital room and Val lays on the bed.

VAL	*(Eats ice cream) [Sign]* I am done. The ice cream was very good.

HUMPHREY   *[Sign]* What do you want to do now?

VAL   *[Sign]* I would like to play checkers with CW. I love checkers.

HUMPHREY   *[Voice]* CW, Val would like to play checkers with you.

CW   *[Sign]* Okay, are you ready to play?

VAL   *[Sign]* Yes.

NURSE   *[Voice as Humphrey signs to Val]* Hello, it is time to take your medicine.

VAL   *[Sign]* No! I don't want it.

HUMPHREY   *[Sign]* It will help you to relax. You will get better.

VAL   *[Sign]* I know, but it makes me very sleepy. I want to play checkers.

NURSE   *[Voice as Humphrey signs to Val]* Sorry, it is important to get better. You can play the game after taking a nap.

HUMPHREY   *[Sign]* I think she is right. It is time for you to take a nap.

VAL   *[Sign]* CW, I am very sorry.

CW   *[Sign]* It is alright. We will play next time.

HUMPHREY   *[Sign]* Are you ready?

VAL   *[Sign]* I guess so.

The nurse puts the shot into Val's IV machine.

VAL   *[Sign]* I feel sleepy.

HUMPHREY   *[Sign]* I know, please relax and take a nap.

Val closes his eyes and falls asleep.

THE NURSE   *[Voice]* He will be alright. Thanks for
                    understanding; have a good day.

CW   *[Voice]* We can stay and relax until his parents
                    arrive. It is time for my nap too.

HUMPHREY   *[Voice]* Okay, I am going to sew something.

Two hours later, Fallon and Betty arrive.

BETTY   *[Voice]* Hello Mary Sue, I am so sorry I woke
                    you up.

HUMPHREY   *[Voice]* It is okay, it has been a long day. Val is
                    still sleeping because the nurse put medicine in
                    his IV. I sewed until I fell sleep.

BETTY   *[Voice]* What were you doing while we were
                    out?

HUMPHREY   *[Voice]* Val ate the hospital food and he realized
                    it tasted the same as at school so he ate it all.
                    The nurse had him take a walk in the hallway,
                    then he asked for ice cream. After, he took
                    some medicine and fell asleep.

BETTY   *[Voice]* Great to hear. Thanks so much for
                    taking care of Val; I appreciate it.

HUMPHREY   *[Voice]* Welcome, anytime.

BETTY   *[Voice]* I'm thinking of getting a tomato garden
                    like yours. Can you tell me how to grow one? I
                    will start it when we get home from the
                    hospital.

HUMPHREY   *[Voice]* I will be glad to tell you. Val told me that tomatoes are your favorite vegetable.

BETTY   *[Voice]* I love them, I use them for fixing salad.

Val wakes up and watches as Humphrey and CW prepare to leave.

VAL   *[Sign]* Humphrey, where are you going? Home?

HUMPHREY   *[Sign]* Yes, we have to go home. Thomas and
                    Blaine are waiting for us.

VAL   *[Sign]* What about playing checkers with CW? I
                    just woke up.

HUMPHREY   *[Sign]* I know, but you can play with him next
                    time. Please understand.

VAL   *[Sign]* I understand. When will I see you again?

HUMPHREY   *[Sign]* We will have to wait and see. *(Hugs Val)*
                    Please take care, I love you. See you later.

VAL   *[Sign]* I love you too, Humphrey. *(Hugs CW)*
                    Thanks so much for coming.

CW   *[Sign]* You are welcome, anytime.

FALLON   *[Voice]* Thanks so much for coming; Val
                    enjoyed the company. Have a safe trip.

BETTY   *(Hugs Humphrey)* *[Voice]* We appreciate you two
                    watching him for us. Please call me when you
                    get home.

HUMPHREY   *[Voice]* Sure, see all of you soon, bye. *(They leave)*

Val watches them leave and cries.

BETTY   *[Sign]* What's wrong, dear?

VAL   *[Sign]* I am very sad to see them leave. They are very sweet and kind; I love them.

BETTY   *[Sign]* You will see them again.

VAL   *[Sign]* When will I see them again?

BETTY   *[Sign]* I don't know.

FALLON   *[Voice]* Betty, come on.

BETTY   *[Voice]* Val looks very upset, what can we do?

FALLON   *[Voice]* Why don't we invite Mary Sue and CW to our house for Val's birthday? I am sure that will make Val very happy.

BETTY   *[Voice]* Good idea! Why don't we tell him now?

FALLON   *[Voice]* Sure, come on.

BETTY   *[Voice]* Please stop them before they leave. I think they are in the lobby now.

FALLON   *[Voice]* Okay, I will go ask them now. *(He leaves)*

VAL   *[Sign]* Why is papa leaving? He seems very excited.

BETTY   *[Sign]* He will be back. Do you want to invite them to come to our house for your birthday?

VAL   *[Sign]* Yes, I want them to come to our house. I want Thomas and Blaine there, too.

BETTY   *[Sign]* Yes, that's why papa left to tell them about your birthday party.

VAL   *(Hugs his mother) [Sign]* Thanks so much Mama; that's what I want for my birthday!

BETTY   *(Laughs) [Sign]* Yes, I know.

Duke Hospital Lobby

Fallon rushes to the lobby and stops Humphrey and her husband from leaving.

FALLON	*[Voice]* Mary Sue! CW! Wait!
HUMPHREY	*[Voice]* Hey Fallon, did I forget something?
FALLON	*[Voice]* No, Betty and I want to invite you to our house for Val's birthday. He will be very happy to see you.
HUMPHREY	*[Voice]* Thanks so much, can Thomas and Blaine come too?
FALLON	*[Voice]* Of course, they are welcome to come. Alan will be home from camp before Val's birthday.
CW	*[Voice]* We would love to go to your house. Can you give us your address?
FALLON	*[Voice]* Don't worry, I will mail the directions.
HUMPHREY	*[Voice]* Okay, we will be there, July 30th right?
FALLON	*[Voice]* That's right.
CW	*[Voice]* Thanks so much, see you then.
HUMPHREY	*(Hugs Fallon) [Voice]* Thanks so much for letting us visit Val here.
FALLON	*[Voice]* Welcome anytime, I know how much Val loves you.
HUMPHREY	*[Voice]* We better go now. We will keep in touch, please call me when Val gets home. Bye.
FALLON	*[Voice]* Sure, thanks. Bye.

July 30, 1977 is Val's 8th birthday

The Humphreys drive to the Melvin residence and find Val and Alan playing on the tire swing.

CW	*[Voice]* We are in Trent Woods. What is the Melvin's address?
HUMPHREY	*[Voice]* 3050 Red Fox road, it is a yellow house.
BLAINE	*[Voice]* Is that Alan and Val? They are on a tire swing.
HUMPHREY	*[Voice]* Yes! That's them! Val loves swinging.
ALAN	*(Looks at them) [Sign]* Val! Your teacher is here! Here they come.

Humphrey's car stops and they get out.

VAL	*(Goes to Mrs. Humphrey and hugs her) [Sign]* Hello Mrs. Humphrey, I am happy to see all of you. Here is my house.
HUMPHREY	*[Sign]* Happy birthday, Val! Your house is nice. I am glad we made it.
VAL	*[Sign]* Thanks so much! I am glad that all of you are here. *(Turns to Alan)* This is Mr. Humphrey and their two sons, Blaine and Thomas.
ALAN	*[Voice]* Hello, Thomas and Blaine! Nice to meet you. Val told me all about you.
BLAINE	*[Voice]* Val told me you are a KISS fan; I am a fan too.
ALAN	*[Voice]* Awesome! Let me get Mama and Papa. I want to tell them you are here. All of you come in.

VAL	*(To Humphrey) [Sign]* Mama has a tomato garden like you.
HUMPHREY	*[Sign]* Really? I would love to see it.
VAL	*[Sign]* Sure, come with me. *(Holds Humphrey's arm and goes to the garden)*
FALLON	*[Voice]* Hello, I'm so glad you made it. Welcome to the Melvin residence. Come in and make yourself comfortable.
BETTY	*[Voice]* Where is Mary Sue?
CW	*[Voice]* Val took her to see your tomato garden. I didn't know you have one too.
BETTY	*[Voice]* Ha! I have been working on it. I got good advice from her.
VAL	*[Sign]* Humphrey, aren't they beautiful?
HUMPHREY	*(Laughs) [Sign]* They are. I think your parents are looking for us.

In the living room at the Melvin's residence, everyone is celebrating Val's birthday.

BETTY	*[Sign]* Val, here is your birthday cake, make a wish.
VAL	*[Sign]* Yes, I have a wish for my birthday.
BETTY	*[Sign]* Tell us what it is.
VAL	*[Sign]* That Mrs. Humphrey will be my teacher again this fall.
HUMPHREY	*(In tears) [Sign]* Oh, Val!
VAL	*[Sign]* You okay, Humphrey?

HUMPHREY   *[Sign]* Yes, you made me cry. I would love to be
                your teacher again.

ALAN   *[Sign]* Are you going to blow out the candles?
                We are ready to eat the cake!

VAL   *[Sign]* I need someone to help me blow out my
                candles.

BETTY   *[Sign]* Okay, who?

VAL   *[Sign]* Humphrey, I need her help.

Everyone looks at Humphrey.

HUMPHREY   *[Sign]* Me?

Val nods his head.

HUMPHREY   *[Sign to Val and voice to his parents]* I am honored
                to help you blow out the candles. *(Turns to
                Fallon and Betty)* Is it okay with you if I help
                him?

BETTY   *[Voice]* Of course, he is waiting for you.

VAL   *[Sign]* Come on, Humphrey!

HUMPHREY   *[Sign]* Okay, I am here with you.

Everyone sings happy birthday to Val.

BETTY   *[Sign and voice]* 1…2…3…Ready!

Val and Mrs. Humphrey blow out the candles as everyone claps their hands.

VAL   *(Hugs Humphrey) [Sign]* Thanks so much. I am
                glad you are here.

HUMPHREY   *[Sign]* You are welcome anytime. Happy
                birthday Val!

They eat cake and ice cream. Val opens his birthday gifts from his family and the Humphrey family. Val thanks them and hugs them. Val and the other boys play outside as the Humphreys and the Melvins relax and talk.

CW	*(Looks at the deer mounted on the wall)* *[Voice]* You hunt deer?
FALLON	*[Voice]* Yes, I've hunted deer my whole life. We eat it sometimes.
CW	*[Voice]* Interesting! Does Val eat it?
FALLON	*[Voice]* No, Val dislikes my hunting deer because he thinks they are Santa's reindeer.
CW	*(Laughs)* *[Voice]* Funny, do you mind if I join you someday?
FALLON	*[Voice]* Yes, do you hunt deer too?
CW	*[Voice]* Yes, I have all my life.
FALLON	*[Voice]* Great, I will check the hunting schedule; then we can decide on a date.
CW	*[Voice]* Sure, thanks.

Betty brings the photo albums of Val as a baby and shows them to Mrs. Humphrey.

BETTY	*[Voice]* Here are baby pictures of Val, I thought you may want to see them.
HUMPHREY	*(Looks at the photo albums)* *[Voice]* He was very cute. I am glad that you and Fallon are able to take care of Val.
BETTY	*[Voice]* Thanks so much. We still love him more than words could ever say.
HUMPHREY	*[Voice]* I am sure you are loving and caring parents. Your letter about his birth was so

	touching. I felt awful for your son.
BETTY	*[Voice]* Oh sorry, I didn't mean to make you feel like that.
HUMPHREY	*[Voice]* It is okay, I am glad you wrote the letter to me. That's when I decided to help him learn.
BETTY	*[Voice]* Wait, the letter made you decide to help Val? That amazes me. I know you didn't give up on him.
HUMPHREY	*[Voice]* We became closer as I taught him.
BETTY	*(Hugs her) [Voice]* I am glad Val had you as a teacher. Thanks so much for caring about him. He has wonderful memories with you. What is your favorite moment with him?
HUMPHREY	*(Laughs) [Voice]* Making him eat pimento cheese sandwiches. He refused to eat them until I put them into his mouth. The he ate it so quickly, I was scared he would choke.
BETTY	*[Voice]* We don't want him to eat quickly because of his jaws.
HUMPHREY	*[Voice]* I know, that's why Val sat next to me at lunch so I could keep an eye on him. Simmons got the dietary staff to prepare soft food for him.
BETTY	*[Voice]* Thanks again, we really appreciate what you did for Val.
FALLON	*[Voice]* Mary Sue, Betty and I have something special for you. Here is a $100 bill. You helped our son learn. We appreciate what you did for him. He is getting better, thanks to you.

HUMPHREY   *[Voice]* Thanks so much, but I can't accept
                your offer. Sorry.

FALLON   *[Voice]* Why?

HUMPHREY   *[Voice]* I don't want your money, Val's love is
                enough of a reward. He is like another son to
                me. Don't worry, we are good friends.

FALLON   *[Voice]* Great to hear. We want you to be part
                of Val's life, but I understand if you don't
                want money from us. It is okay.

HUMPHREY   *[Voice]* Thanks so much for understanding. We
                can keep in touch in the future. CW and I are
                going to build a cottage in Pamlico County.
                We want all of you to come there one day.

FALLON   *[Voice]* Wow, I preached there, before we
                moved to Riverdale last year. Where is your
                cottage located?

CW   *[Voice]* In Oriental. Have you been there?

FALLON   *[Voice]* Yes, I preached at churches in small
                towns. The people are sweet and kind. Val met
                a deaf man in Stonewall, his name was Asa
                Gatlin Jr.

HUMPHREY   *[Voice]* Is he still alive?

FALLON   *[Voice]* No, he died last year. Val is too young
                to understand death. I told him that Asa had
                to go to heaven to be with the Lord.

BETTY   *[Voice]* Mary Sue, we need to talk to you about
                something important.

HUMPHREY   *[Voice]* Sure what is it?

BETTY   *[Voice]* I am glad Val asked you to teach him again, we also want you to. You did an amazing job with him. Do you think Simmons will let you continue to teach him?

HUMPHREY   *[Voice]* I will discuss it with Simmons.

FALLON   *[Voice]* Great! Please call us after the discussion.

HUMPHREY   *[Voice]* Sure, I will.

Outside the Melvin Residence

CW and Humphrey get ready to go home. They go outside to find the kids playing on the tire swing.

CW   *[Voice]* Boys, it is time to go home.

BLAINE   *[Voice]* I enjoy the tire swing, it is so much fun.

THOMAS   *[Voice]* Me too, but I need to go, and I am meeting someone tonight.

HUMPHREY   *[Voice]* Right, say goodbye to Val and his family. We will see them again.

VAL   *[Sign]* Are you leaving now? I am sad.

HUMPHREY   *[Sign]* Please don't be sad. We will get together in the school year. Okay?

VAL   *[Sign]* Okay, thanks so much for coming over. I love your gift.

HUMPHREY   *[Sign]* You are welcome. I will see you at school next month. I love you.

VAL   *[Sign]* I love you too. Wait.

HUMPHREY   *[Sign]* Yes?

VAL	*[Sign]* Don't forget to tell Simmons that you want to teach me again.
HUMPHREY	*[Sign]* Sure, I won't.
BETTY	*(Hugs Humphrey)* *[Voice]* Thanks so much Mary Sue. We enjoyed having you and your family. We will be glad to visit your cottage when it is finished.
HUMPHREY	*[Voice]* Sure, no problem. Your garden is beautiful. Thanks, see you later.
CW	*[Voice]* Call me when you are ready to go deer hunting.
FALLON	*[Voice]* Got it. Please be safe driving home.

Humphrey's car starts and leaves as the Melvin family waves goodbye.

ALAN	*[Voice]* Mrs. Humphrey is an amazing teacher. Do you think she will teach Val again?
FALLON	*[Voice]* I hope so.

Scene Seventeen: "Humphrey is Not Your Teacher Anymore."

The Eagles Hall Lunchroom

The teachers go to the lunchroom for a meeting with Simmons about the new school year. Humphrey is very pleased to come back to the school and see her best friend, Beth Dawson.

DAWSON	*[Voice]* Hello Humphrey, I can't believe the summer is almost over, but it is great to be here. How was it?
HUMPHREY	*[Voice]* It was very good and busy. I saw Val three times this summer, he is doing fine.

DAWSON   *[Voice]* I heard that he was in the hospital. What happened?

HUMPHREY   *[Voice]* It was just his ear operation. The doctor reshaped his ears so he can wear his hearing aids. I need to talk to Simmons before the meeting.

DAWSON   *[Voice]* Really, what is it?

HUMPHREY   *[Voice]* I would like to keep Val as my student for another year. I enjoyed having him.

DAWSON   *[Voice]* Before you go talk to Simmons, you should know that she already made the student list for us.

HUMPHREY   *[Voice]* Will Val be my student again?

DAWSON   *[Voice]* Uh-oh, I don't know, but wait and see.

Simmons shows up and asks everyone to sit down. The discussion begins.

SIMMONS   *[Voice]* Good morning teachers, welcome back to work. I was very impressed with your teaching, you did an amazing job last year, but this year will be a little different. I hope you don't mind that. I have the student list for you.

HUMPHREY   *(Sighs)* *[Voice]* Here we go.

SIMMONS   *[Voice]* Teachers, are you all ready for the student list?

The teachers nod their heads.

SIMMONS   *[Voice]* Here it is. *(Gives the student list to each teacher as Humphrey closes her eyes)*

DAWSON   *[Voice]* Humphrey, why did you close your eyes?

HUMPHREY   *[Voice]* I want to be surprised. Is it here?

DAWSON   *(Clears her throat)* *[Voice]* Yes, it is. Open your eyes.

HUMPHREY   *(Opens her eyes and reads the list)* *[Voice]* Ah, no!

DAWSON   *[Voice]* Ugh! It's bad news, I am so sorry.

Humphrey gets upset and goes to Simmons' office.

HUMPHREY   *[Voice]* Simmons, may I talk to you for a minute?

SIMMONS   *[Voice]* Sure, we can talk. I know why you look upset, Val is not on your list. I put him in the first grade.

HUMPHREY   *[Voice]* First grade?

SIMMONS   *[Voice]* Yes, his grade had improved so I moved him to the next level with his classmates.

HUMPHREY   *[Voice]* You mean the classmates I taught?

SIMMONS   *[Voice]* That's right. They are now in the first grade in Eatmon's class. I know you want to teach him again, but it is time to move on.

HUMPHREY   *[Voice]* Clara Eatmon is Val's next teacher?

SIMMONS   *[Voice]* Yes, she is. I am sure she will teach him as well as you did. I know it is hard for you, but it is time for Val to have a different teacher.

HUMPHREY   *[Voice]* Val and I became closer when he spent a week with me and my family. We visited him in the hospital, and he invited us to come to his house for his birthday. It made me feel

	very close to him and made me want to teach him again.
SIMMONS	*[Voice]* I know how you feel about Val. Did he ask you if you would teach him again?
HUMPHREY	*[Voice]* Yes, he got very excited when he asked me at his birthday party. His parents want me to teach him again too. They want me to be a part of his life.
SIMMONS	*[Voice]* I understand, you are a part of his life. You are not his teacher anymore, but you can see him sometimes. I know his parents are very impressed with what you did for Val.
HUMPHREY	*[Voice]* Thanks, Simmons. What about Eatmon?
SIMMONS	*[Voice]* Well, we are going to discuss Val so she will know what to do for him. I am sure she will do the same thing for him that you did. Please do me a favor.
HUMPHREY	*[Voice]* Val will be heartbroken when he finds out. What is it?
SIMMONS	*[Voice]* Call his parents and tell them that you are not his teacher anymore. Remind them to tell Val about his new teacher. Let's go see Eatmon and talk to her. Come with me.
HUMPHREY	*(Clears her throat)* *[Voice]* Okay, I understand, but I don't want to upset him.
SIMMONS	*[Voice]* Val will be alright. He will get over it.

The Living Room at the Melvin Residence

In the Melvin residence, Betty gets the bad news from Mrs. Humphrey and is heartbroken. Fallon sees her in tears.

FALLON   *[Voice]* What's wrong dear? You look upset.

BETTY   *[Voice]* I got a call from Mary Sue. She informed me that she is not Val's teacher this year. His new teacher is Clara Eatmon.

FALLON   *[Voice]* Oh no, I thought she wanted to teach him again. What happened?

BETTY   *[Voice]* Simmons made the student list for the teachers, but Val is not on Humphrey's list. She is heartbroken.

FALLON   *[Voice]* I understand, but we will talk to her about putting Val back with Humphrey.

BETTY   *[Voice]* We can't do that. She put him in the first grade.

FALLON   *[Voice]* First grade? I am very happy and proud of him. Do we tell him?

BETTY   *[Voice]* I am very happy for him too, but disappointed for Humphrey. She asked us not to tell him until he comes back to school. I want to see him very happy.

FALLON   *[Voice]* Me too, wait and see.

Val and his parents go to Eagles Hall for the start of the new school year. Val is excited to be there, but he still has no idea that he will have a different teacher.

The Foyer

VAL   *(Gets excited) [Sign]* Mrs. Cole! I am very happy to see you! *(Hugs Mrs. Cole)* Missed you lots!

COLE   *[Sign]* I am happy to see you, I missed you too.

How was your summer?

VAL

[Sign] I had fun with Humphrey. I thought of you when I got your birthday card, thanks so much for the money.

COLE

[Sign] You are welcome anytime. I heard you went to the hospital, but I am glad you are better.

VAL

[Sign] Yes, I am fine. Here are some tomatoes for you. Mama grew them in her garden.

COLE

[Sign to Val and voice to his parents] Aww sweet, thanks so much. *(Turns to Val's parents)* Hello Mr. and Mrs. Melvin. Thanks so much for the tomatoes.

BETTY

[Voice] You are welcome; I am glad you like them.

COLE

[Voice] You okay? You look a little upset.

FALLON

[Voice] We got a message from Humphrey, Val got a different teacher this year. He doesn't know yet, but he will find out soon.

COLE

[Voice] Look at him, he is very excited to be here.

BETTY

[Voice] Until he finds out Humphrey is not his teacher.

COLE

[Voice] Aw, poor Val. I will comfort him with cake and milk.

BETTY

[Voice] Thanks so much, I am glad that you two are very close. See you later.

The Middle of Eagles Hall

Val and his parents walk down the hallway and find Simmons.

SIMMONS   *[Voice]* Good afternoon, Mr. and Mrs. Melvin.
                   I am happy to see you, it is great to see Val
                   very happy.

FALLON   *[Voice]* Thanks, Val is excited to be back.

SIMMONS   *(Looks at Val) [Sign]* That sounds great. You
                   have an apple for your teacher?

VAL   *[Sign]* Yes, it is for Mrs. Humphrey. I am very
                   happy to have her as my teacher again.

SIMMONS   *(Looks a little upset) [Sign to Val and voice to his
                   parents]* That's very sweet. *(Turns to Val's
                   parents)* You didn't tell him that Humphrey is
                   not his teacher?

*Val's parents look at each other and shake their heads. They don't say
anything.*

SIMMONS   *[Voice]* Got it, we will talk about it later.

*After registration, Val and his parents go to the dorm to leave his suitcase on
his bed. They go down the hallway to Eatmon's classroom.*

EATMON   *[Voice]* Good afternoon! You must be the
                   parents of Val Melvin.

FALLON   *[Voice]* Nice to meet you, Eatmon. My name is
                   Fallon Melvin and this is my wife Betty. I am
                   sure our son will enjoy your class.

EATMON   *[Voice]* I am very happy to have him as my
                   student. Humphrey told me everything about
                   him. Where is he? I haven't seen him.

BETTY   *(Looks around) [Voice]* Fallon, have you seen
                   Val?

FALLON   *[Voice]* I think he went to see Mrs. Humphrey. He still thinks she is his teacher again. We need to get him.

BETTY   *[Voice]* Eatmon, I am very sorry. We will be back, alright?

EATMON   *[Voice]* It is okay. See you later.

Humphrey's Classroom

Val goes to Humphrey's classroom and is excited to see her.

VAL   *(Hugs Humphrey)* *[Sign]* I am very happy to see you. Here is an apple for you because you are my teacher again.

HUMPHREY   *[Sign]* How sweet! I know how you feel, but I have to tell you something.

Val's parents show up.

BETTY   *[Voice]* Hello Humphrey, we just met Val's new teacher, and we need to take him to meet Eatmon now.

HUMPHREY   *[Voice]* Please wait, I need to tell him something. I want you to stay with us so you can comfort him.

BETTY   *[Voice]* Good idea, he will be heartbroken.

FALLON   *[Voice]* It is time to tell him the truth. We are here with you.

HUMPHREY   *[Voice to parents and sign to Val]* Thanks so much, I appreciate it. *(Turns to Val)* Val, I have to tell you something, please listen to me carefully.

VAL   *[Sign]* Okay, tell me.

Simmons shows up and finds Val and his parents in Humphrey's classroom.

SIMMONS	*(Sounds upset)* *[Voice]* Hey Mr. and Mrs. Melvin, I thought you were supposed to meet Val's new teacher. What are you doing here?
FALLON	*[Voice]* Take it easy, we already met her, but Val came here to see Humphrey. He still thinks she is his teacher. She is ready to tell him the truth.
SIMMONS	*[Voice]* Well, I need to talk to Humphrey now. Please take Val to the dorm and unpack his clothes. You can come back later.
BETTY	*[Voice]* But…
SIMMONS	*[Voice]* Please go to the dorm, now.
FALLON	*[Voice to Betty and sign to Val]* We have to listen to her because she is the principal. *(Turns to Val)* We need to unpack your clothes, but we will be back. Okay?
VAL	*[Sign]* Okay, see you later.

Val and his parents leave.

HUMPHREY	*[Voice]* Simmons, why did you do that to them? I was supposed to tell him that I am not his teacher anymore, but you interrupted.
SIMMONS	*[Voice]* You asked his parents not to tell Val that you are no longer his teacher?
HUMPHREY	*[Voice]* I don't want him to be disappointed.
SIMMONS	*[Voice]* I know what you mean, but he will get over it.
HUMPHREY	*[Voice]* Take it easy, please don't give him a

	hard time in front of his parents. We need a chance to tell him.
SIMMONS	[Voice] That's it, we can tell him after his parents leave.
HUMPHREY	[Voice] You are going to get rid of them?
SIMMONS	[Voice] I don't mean it like that, but I will explain everything to them. I am sure they will understand.
HUMPHREY	[Voice] I don't want Val to get hurt.
SIMMONS	[Voice] I think you spend too much time with him. That's why he wants you to teach him again.
HUMPHREY	(Gets mad) [Voice] Okay! You win!
FALLON	[Voice] Hello Miss Simmons, we are back. We have unpacked everything and are ready for you to tell Val.
SIMMONS	[Voice] Good, I would like to talk to you two in private if you don't mind.
FALLON	[Voice] I don't mind. What is it about?
SIMMONS	[Voice] Go to the hallway, and I will tell you.
BETTY	[Voice] Okay, what about Val?
SIMMONS	[Voice] He can stay with Humphrey while we talk in the hallway. Let's go there.
BETTY	[Sign] Val, please stay with Humphrey. We will have a talk with Miss Simmons. We will be back soon, okay?
VAL	[Sign] Okay.

The Class Hallway

Simmons has a talk with Val's parents outside Humphrey's classroom.

FALLON   *[Voice]* What do you want to talk about? We
                  need to tell Val about his next teacher and we
                  need to comfort him if he is upset.

BETTY   *[Voice]* I agree with my husband.

SIMMONS   *[Voice]* I understand and I don't blame you for
                  that, but I think it is best to tell Val after you
                  leave.

FALLON   *[Voice]* You want us to leave now?

SIMMONS   *[Voice]* Yes, I think it would be best. I don't
                  want him to run to you when we tell him
                  about his new teacher. That's why I'm asking
                  you to leave. I hope you won't be angry.

BETTY   *(Gets mad) [Voice]* No way! We need to be here
                  to comfort him if he needs us.

SIMMONS   *[Voice]* Mrs. Melvin…

FALLON   *[Voice]* Hold on, Miss Simmons. *(Turns to his
                  wife)* Betty, she is right. It is her job to help Val
                  accept his new teacher. We will let her do this.

BETTY   *[Voice]* Simmons, you are right. Are you sure
                  you can do it?

SIMMONS   *[Voice]* Of course, don't worry. He will be
                  alright. I will call you if something happens.
                  Thanks so much for understanding.

BETTY   *[Voice]* Thanks so much. May we have time to
                  say goodbye to him before we leave?

SIMMONS   *[Voice]* Sure, no problem.

Humphrey's Classroom

Simmons and Val's parents come back into the classroom. Humphrey looks nervous because Simmons is not pleased with her.

SIMMONS	*[Voice to Humphrey and sign to Val]* They understand, they have to leave now. Val, you can go with your parents and say goodbye. Come back here when they leave.
VAL	*[Sign]* Okay. Humphrey, I will be back.
BETTY	*[Voice]* It was very nice to see you Humphrey. I am so sorry about today.
HUMPHREY	*[Voice]* It is okay. I will see him sometimes. Please be safe, take care.
BETTY	*[Voice]* You too, bye.

They leave and say goodbye to Val.

Later, Val comes back to Humphrey's classroom.

VAL	*[Sign]* Hello, I am back. I didn't cry when my parents left, I am very happy here.
SIMMONS	*[Sign]* I am happy for you. I want you to read the student list on Humphrey's door.
VAL	*[Sign]* Am I on the list?
SIMMONS	*(Points to the door)* *[Sign]* Please read the list.
VAL	*(Goes to the door and reads the list)* *[Sign]* I am not in Humphrey's class. Why?
SIMMONS	*[Sign]* You have to move to another classroom. Your new teacher is Clara Eatmon. She teaches first grade.

VAL   *[Sign]* What about Humphrey? I asked her to teach me again.

HUMPHREY   *[Voice]* Simmons...

SIMMONS   *[Voice to Humphrey and sign to Val]* Please let me handle him. *(Turns to Val)* Humphrey teaches kindergarten. She is not your teacher anymore. It is time to meet your new teacher, Mrs. Eatmon.

VAL   *[Sign]* Humphrey, you don't want to teach me again?

HUMPHREY   *[Sign]* I would love to teach you again, but you are in the first grade now. You have the same classmates. Please accept Mrs. Eatmon as your teacher.

VAL   *[Sign]* No way! I want you to teach me again.

HUMPHREY   *(Turns to Simmons)* *[Voice]* I don't know what to do.

SIMMONS   *(Ignores her and turns to Val)* *[Sign]* Come with me Val, we need to go meet your teacher and get to know her.

VAL   *[Sign]* No! I am staying here.

SIMMONS   *(Gets mad and spanks his butt)* *[Sign]* You're a bad boy! *(Val cries)*

HUMPHREY   *[Voice]* Simmons! Don't do that!

SIMMONS   *[Voice to Humphrey and sign to Val]* You are not his teacher anymore! *(Turns to Val)* Go to Mrs. Eatmon classroom, now! *(Simmons grabs Val's arm and pulls him away from the classroom as Humphrey looks on and cries)*

The Class Hallway

The next morning, Val walks in the class hallway to go to Mrs. Humphrey's classroom, but the door is locked. He knocks on the door hard until Simmons shows up.

SIMMONS	*[Sign]* Val, what are you doing here? You are supposed to go to Eatmon's class.
VAL	*[Sign]* I wanted to say good morning to Mrs. Humphrey, that's all.
SIMMONS	*[Sign]* She is not your teacher anymore! Go to Eatmon's classroom now!
VAL	*(Ignores Simmons)* *[Sign]* I want to see her, now.
SIMMOMS	*(Gets mad and spanks his butt, hard)* *[Sign]* Go!

Val cries and is forced to go to Eatmon's classroom. Mrs. Humphrey hears his cry.

The Eagles Hall Lunchroom

Clara Eatmon and the students sit at the circle table. They eat pimento cheese sandwiches and vegetable soup. They remind Val of Humphrey.

EATMON	*[Sign]* Val, please eat your lunch.
VAL	*[Sign]* No way!
EATMON	*(Sighs)* *[Sign]* I am going to get Humphrey.
SIMMONS	*(Goes to the table and looks at Val)* *[Voice]* Mrs. Eatmon, don't do that. Please make him eat.
EATMON	*[Voice]* Why not?
SIMMONS	*[Voice]* She is not his teacher anymore, you are and he is your student.

EATMON	*[Voice]* What if he doesn't eat lunch?
SIMMONS	*[Voice]* Put him in the corner.
VAL	*[Sign]* Eatmon, may I ask you something?
EATMON	*[Sign]* Sure, ask me anything.
VAL	*[Sign]* Can I eat lunch with Mrs. Humphrey please?

Eatmon gasps and looks at Simmons, then turns to Val who is mad.

EATMON	*[Sign]* No, you have to stay with us. She is not your teacher anymore, I am your teacher now.
VAL	*[Sign]* Okay, I will stay here, but I am not going to eat.
EATMON	*[Sign]* Val, you will be hungry soon.
VAL	*[Sign]* I will drink milk.
EATMON	*(Pulls the milk from him) [Sign]* No milk for you until you eat your lunch.
VAL	*(Gets up) [Sign]* I am going to leave now.
EATMON	*(Grabs him and puts him on the chair) [Sign]* No! Val, stay here!
SIMMONS	*[Voice]* Well, I will take him to my office and put him in the corner.
EATMON	*[Voice]* I guess he doesn't listen to what I say.
SIMMONS	*(Grabs Val's arm) [Sign]* Val, please come with me to my office.
CINDY	*[Sign]* Traci, Val is back to his old ways. What can we do?

TRACI   *[Sign]* I better get Humphrey to talk to him. Be
                 back soon.

SIMMONS   *[Sign]* Traci! Where are you going?

TRACI   *[Sign]* You will find out. *(She walks to Humphrey)*
                 Humphrey, I think you need to talk to Val and
                 make him accept Eatmon as his teacher.

HUMPHREY   *[Sign]* Traci, I want to talk to him, but I can't.

TRACI   *[Sign]* I know, but you taught him
                 kindergarten. Please talk to him. You are very
                 close to each other and he needs you now.

HUMPHREY   *(Gets up)* *[Sign]* Okay, I will try my best. *(Turns
                 to her students)* Please behave yourselves. I have
                 to talk to Val, I will be back.

Humphrey and Traci go to Eatmon's table.

TRACI   *[Sign]* Simmons, please let Humphrey talk to
                 Val, he always listens to her.

SIMMONS   *[Sign and voice]* Okay, good luck!

HUMPHREY   *[Sign]* Val, please listen to me, I need to talk to
                 you. I am sad that you don't accept Eatmon as
                 your teacher. I told her about you and she will
                 do the same things for you that I did.

VAL   *[Sign]* I know, but nobody replaces you. Why
                 did Simmons change my teacher?

HUMPHREY   *[Sign]* It is her job to change the student list for
                 teachers every year. I got upset, but I have to
                 accept it. I have to tell you something about
                 Eatmon.

VAL   *[Sign]* Really, what is it?

HUMPHREY   *[Sign]* You and Eatmon have the same
                    birthday: July 30th.

VAL   *[Sign]* Really? *(Turns to Eatmon)* July 30th is your
                    birthday too?

EATMON   *[Sign]* Right, we have the same birthday. I tried
                    to tell you, but you didn't listen to me.

VAL   *[Sign]* I am so sorry I was mean to you. It is
                    very nice to have the same birthday.

EATMON   *[Sign]* No problem, thanks.

VAL   *[Sign]* Eatmon, I accept you as my teacher.
                    That's what Humphrey wants. Is it okay if I
                    hug you?

EATMON   *(Hugs Val)* *[Sign]* Thanks, please listen to what
                    I say.

VAL   *[Sign]* Okay, I will do that.

EATMON   *[Sign]* Thanks again, you better eat lunch now.

VAL   *[Sign]* Okay. *(Eats his lunch)* Thanks Humphrey;
                    Eatmon is very happy now.

EATMON   *[Voice]* Thanks, Humphrey, I appreciate your
                    help. It means a lot to me.

HUMPHREY   *[Voice]* Welcome, anytime. I better go back to
                    my table, bye.

EATMON   *[Voice]* Wait.

HUMPHREY   *[Voice]* Yes?

EATMON   *(Turns to Val)* *[Sign]* I know you are sad that
                    Humphrey is not your teacher anymore, but
                    you were lucky to have her, you can give her a

big hug if you want.

VAL   *[Sign]* Okay, can I see her sometimes?

EATMON   *[Sign]* Yes, she is still special to you because she loves you. I know you two are very close.

VAL   *[Sign]* Humphrey, please don't be sad, *(Hugs her)* I will see you sometimes, and I will never forget you.

HUMPHREY   *[Sign]* Oh Val, I love you. Please obey Eatmon.

VAL   *[Sign]* Yes, I will. I love you too.

Eatmon smiles and winks at Humphrey.

The kids are excited and raise their arms in congratulations.

SIMMONS   *[Voice]* Wow! That was amazing. The problem is solved.

The Eagles Hall Foyer

In August 1978, Humphrey arrives at Eagles Hall. Cole sees her in the foyer.

COLE   *[Voice]* Hey, Humphrey!

HUMPHREY   *[Voice]* Hello, Mrs. Cole.

COLE   *[Voice]* I have to tell you something important about Val.

HUMPHREY   *[Voice]* Is everything alright with him? You look very sad.

COLE   *[Voice]* Yes, I am sad. He is doing fine, but he is no longer staying at Eagles Hall. He moved to Vestal Hall for the second grade.

HUMPHREY	*[Voice]* Aw, I am going to miss him. Who is his teacher?
COLE	*[Voice]* Her name is Sue Dail; she is very sweet like you.
HUMPHREY	*[Voice]* Really? I am going to check up on him after school. Thanks, I miss him so much.
COLE	*[Voice]* Me too. Eagles Hall is not the same without him. Please keep in touch with Val and his family.
HUMPHREY	*[Voice]* Sure, thanks. I will never forget him and his family.

Scene Eighteen: The News of Grandpa's Death

In March, 1979, on a snowy night, Humphrey feels bad that Val has to spend the weekend in the dorm. She gets a call from Betty who informs her that her father passed away. She wants Val to spend the weekend with Humphrey so she can comfort him. Humphrey accepts Betty's wish.

Humphrey Residence

CW	*[Voice]* Mary Sue, what's wrong? You look upset.
HUMPHREY	*[Voice]* I got a call from Betty, she informed me that her father passed away yesterday.
CW	*[Voice]* I am very sorry to hear about that. Does Val know about his grandpa?
HUMPHREY	*[Voice]* He doesn't know yet, she asked me if he could spend the weekend with us, so I could comfort him.
CW	*[Voice]* Why don't his parents pick him up? He

	needs to be with his family, especially his grandmother.
HUMPHREY	*[Voice]* They were unable to pick him up due to the weather. They are in Fayetteville with Betty's mother. Fayetteville got a lot of snow.
CW	*[Voice]* Poor Val, why don't we bring him here to be with us?
HUMPHREY	*[Voice]* Of course, I will call the dorm to let them know we will pick Val up.
CW	*[Voice]* The boys are hanging out with their friends. We can write a note so they know where we are.
HUMPHREY	*[Voice]* Okay, let's pick Val up.

Humphrey goes to the boys' dorm in Vestal Hall and finds Val laying on the bed. She hugs him.

HUMPHREY	*[Sign]* Hello Val, it is me. I am here with you.
VAL	*(Wakes up and hugs Humphrey) [Sign]* Humphrey, it is very good to see you. Mama and Papa didn't pick me up today, I need to know why.
HUMPHREY	*[Sign]* Because the roads are dangerous. We are here to take you to our house. Is it okay with you? Your parents want you to stay with us.
VAL	*[Sign]* Okay, I want to stay at your place. I don't want to stay here for the weekend.
HUMPHREY	*[Sign]* Good boy, come on and let's pack your clothes for the weekend.
VAL1	*[Sign]* Thanks for the invite, I feel better.

CW and Humphrey take Val to their place. Val is very pleased to spend the weekend with them.

HUMPHREY	*[Voice]* Boys! We are home. Val is here to spend the weekend with us.
VAL	*(Hugs the boys) [Sign]* Thomas! Blaine! Great to see you two; I am excited to stay with all of you this weekend. I am hungry.
BLAINE	*[Sign]* We are happy to have you here. Here are pimento cheese sandwiches and chocolate milk for you.
THOMAS	*[Sign]* Make yourself comfortable, you are home.
VAL	*[Sign]* Thanks so much. *(He goes to the table and eats the sandwiches)* They are very good.
HUMPHREY	*[Voice]* Boys, how sweet of you. You made him very happy. I appreciate what you do for him.
THOMAS	*[Voice]* We wanted to see him happy. When will you tell him about his grandpa? He will be heartbroken.
HUMPHREY	*[Voice]* Not now, I am going to call his mother and figure out the best time to tell him.
CW	*[Voice]* Mary Sue, where will Val sleep? The sewing room is a mess.
HUMPHREY	*[Voice]* He will sleep on the couch.
THOMAS	*[Voice]* Wait a minute, why don't I let him sleep on my bed while I sleep on the couch?
HUMPHREY	*[Voice]* How sweet of you, he will be more comfortable sleeping there. Blaine, do you mind that?

BLAINE	*[Voice]* I don't mind. Does he snore?
HUMPHREY	*[Voice]* Blaine!
BLAINE	*[Voice]* Take it easy, Mom. I am just kidding. He is welcome to sleep with me.
VAL	*[Sign]* I finished eating the pimento cheese sandwiches. They were very good. *(Turns to the boys)* Thanks so much.
BLAINE	*[Sign]* Welcome anytime. I am glad you liked it.
THOMAS	*[Sign]* You can sleep on my bed if you want. I will sleep on the couch.
VAL	*[Sign]* Wow, how nice of you. Thanks.
HUMPHREY	*[Sign]* Val, I am going to call your mother and let her know you are safe with us. What would you like me to tell her?
VAL	*[Sign]* Tell her I love her, Papa, and Alan and that I miss them, but I am happy to stay with you this weekend.
HUMPHREY	*[Sign]* Good, I will be glad to tell her for you. It is time for you to brush your teeth. Use the boys' bathroom.
VAL	*[Sign]* Okay, what about cleaning my trach?
HUMPHREY	*[Sign]* I will help you later. Okay?
VAL	*[Sign]* Okay. *(He goes to the bathroom)*
CW	*[Voice]* Doesn't he know his parents and Alan are in Fayetteville?
HUMPHREY	*[Voice]* I will explain to him later. *(Dials the number)* Hello Betty, it is me, Mary Sue.

BETTY   *[Voice]* Hello Mary Sue, great to hear from you. Is Val safe with you and your family?

HUMPHREY   *[Voice]* Yes, he is here with us. I explained to him why you didn't pick him up, he understands.

BETTY   *[Voice]* Great to hear. Thanks so much for letting Val stay with you. How is he doing now?

HUMPHREY   *[Voice]* He is doing fine. He is brushing his teeth now. I will clean his trach soon and he will sleep in Thomas' bed. I need to know when we can tell him about his grandpa.

BETTY   *[Voice]* I think tomorrow morning is better, he needs a good night's sleep.

HUMPHREY   *[Voice]* I agree with you. Don't worry, we will take care of him for you. You need to be with your mother, I am sorry about Val not being there. Val said he loves you, Papa, and Alan and he misses all of you!

BETTY   *[Voice]* Thanks so much, we appreciate what you do for him. I will call you before the funeral at ten. Please give Val our love.

HUMPHREY   *[Voice]* Sure, no problem. Please take it easy and tell Alan we are so sorry to hear about your loss and the boys will take care of Val for him. Talk to you tomorrow. Good night and love all of you, bye.

BETTY   *[Voice]* Thanks so much, good night.

VAL   *[Sign]* Was that my mother? What did she say?

HUMPHREY   *[Sign]* Yes, it was her. They couldn't pick you up because the roads are dangerous. It is best for you to stay here. They are at Fayetteville with your grandparents.

VAL

[Sign] Why are they with Grandma and Grandpa?

HUMPHREY

[Sign] They wanted to visit them to check on how they are doing.

VAL

[Sign] Where is Alan?

HUMPHREY

[Sign] He is with them.

VAL

[Sign] Why didn't they get me?

HUMPHREY

[Sign] They wanted to pick you up, but the news warned them about the dangerous road, it is very icy. That's why you will stay with us.

VAL

(Sounds upset) [Sign] It is not fair! I want to see Grandma and Grandpa!

HUMPHREY

[Sign] I know, but they want you to stay here for safety reasons. You will see them soon. Please don't be mad, it is best for you to stay here. They said they love you.

VAL

[Sign] Okay, I miss them.

HUMPHREY

(Hugs Val) [Sign] I know you miss them. They love you.

In the morning, Val eats Rice Krispies and a banana for breakfast as Humphrey waits for his mother to call her. The phone rings and Humphrey answers it.

HUMPHREY

[Voice] Hello, this is the Humphrey residence.

BETTY

[Voice] Hello, Mary Sue, we are getting ready for the funeral. How is Val doing?

HUMPHREY	*[Voice]* Doing fine. I will tell him when he is done with his breakfast.
BETTY	*[Voice]* I know he will be heartbroken. Please be strong, and I want to thank you for letting him stay there. I need to get ready, but I will call you after the funeral. Okay?
HUMPHREY	*[Voice]* Okay, I will tell him. Let me know how the funeral goes. Talk to you later, bye.
CW	*[Voice]* How are Betty and her family doing?
HUMPHREY	*[Voice]* They are doing okay, but very sad. Today is the funeral. I am waiting for Val to finish breakfast to tell him.
CW	*[Voice]* You are right about him, he is like another son to us.
HUMPHREY	*[Voice]* What are you doing today?
CW	*[Voice]* I need to stay here and comfort him.
HUMPHREY	*[Voice]* Here he comes.
VAL	*[Sign]* I am done with my breakfast and put the bowl and spoon in your sink. I need to clean my teeth.
HUMPHREY	*[Sign]* Not now, I have to tell you something important. Please sit down next to me.

Blaine and Thomas show up.

HUMPHREY	*[Voice]* I thought you were going to see your friends?
BLAINE	*[Voice]* We changed our minds, we need to be here for Val. We love him.

THOMAS	*[Voice]* We don't want him to feel lonely. That's why we are here for him
HUMPHREY	*[Voice]* Thanks so much, it is time to tell him about his grandfather.
VAL	*[Sign]* What's going on?
HUMPHREY	*[Sign]* We have important news. Your parents and Alan went to Fayetteville to visit Grandma and Grandpa because Grandpa was very sick.
VAL	*[Sign]* What's wrong with him?
HUMPHREY	*[Sign]* He was ready to go to heaven to be with the Lord. He said he loves you.
VAL	*[Sign]* Is he leaving us?
HUMPHREY	*[Sign]* Yes, he died two days ago. Today is his funeral, they have to bury him.
VAL	*(Cries) [Sign]* I need to go see my family!
HUMPHREY	*(Comforts Val) [Sign]* I know you want to see them, but you have to stay here with us.
VAL	*[Sign]* When will I see Grandpa again?
HUMPHREY	*[Sign]* Someday, he is watching over you. He loves you.
VAL	*[Sign]* Who will take care of Grandma?
HUMPHREY	*[Sign]* Your mother and your aunts will stay with her until she is strong enough to stay alone. She will be fine. I am sure she is thinking of you.

Val starts to cry while Humphrey holds him. Val goes to the bedroom to lay on Thomas' bed.

CW   *[Voice]* Is Val okay?

HUMPHREY   *[Voice]* He's not good, please give him time. He needs to relax.

CW   *[Voice]* Okay, tell me about his grandpa.

HUMPHREY   *[Voice]* His name was Thomas Maurice Woodburn, he was a Sergeant in World War II. He had three daughters and lived in Germany for a while. He enjoyed fishing and spoiled Val with milkshakes.

CW   *[Voice]* He must have been a hero. How did he die?

HUMPHREY   *[Voice]* Skin cancer, he loved smoking like you.

CW   *[Voice]* I know Val is very close to his grandpa. You met both grandparents when Val was in your class?

HUMPHREY   *[Voice]* Right, they visited our classroom. Betty didn't feel well, so she asked them to pick him up instead. Her mother brought some cookies for the students.

CW   *[Voice]* Did she bake the apple pie for us?

HUMPHREY   *[Voice]* She did, because she wanted to thank me for teaching Val.

CW   *[Voice]* She sounds like a sweet lady. Are Fallon's parents alive?

HUMPHREY   *[Voice]* No, his father died a few months before Val was born; his mother died when Val was four. Val hardly remembers his paternal grandmother, but Fallon has a brother named Lewis.

CW   *[Voice]* How rough on him. He has one
                      grandparent left. Val is welcome to come to
                      our house anytime.

HUMPHREY   *[Voice]* Right, well there is not much we can do
                      now. I better wash Val's dirty clothes.

CW   *[Voice]* Let me know if Val needs us.

HUMPHREY   *[Voice]* Sure.

Humphrey removes Val's dirty clothes from the suitcase and puts them into
the washer. A picture falls out of Val's pocket. Humphrey looks at it.

CW   *[Voice]* Dear, what's wrong?

HUMPHREY   *(Looks at the picture) [Voice]* Look at this picture,
                      it is Grandpa and Val. He is wearing a funny
                      hat to make him laugh.

CW   *[Voice]* It's a good picture of them.

HUMPHREY   *[Voice]* Yes, it is, I better take the picture to
                      him.

CW   *[Voice]* Okay, let him know we will go out to
                      eat at the steakhouse for dinner.

HUMPHREY   *[Voice]* Val can't eat steak.

CW   *[Voice]* I know, but you said he can eat
                      meatloaf.

HUMPHREY   *[Voice]* Right, I will tell him.

Humphrey goes to her sons' bedroom and sees Val lying on the bed.
Humphrey sits on the bed and hugs Val.

Humphrey's Boys' Bedroom

HUMPHREY   *[Sign]* You okay Val?

VAL   *(Cries)* *[Sign]* Not good, I am still thinking of
                Grandpa. I am very sad I was not there.

HUMPHREY   *(Gives the picture to Val)* *[Sign]* I know, but I
                found a picture of you and Grandpa.

VAL   *[Sign]* Grandpa!

HUMPHREY   *[Sign]* I know you are sad, so my husband
                wants to take us to eat out.

VAL   *[Sign]* I am not hungry.

HUMPHREY   *[Sign]* You need to eat. Grandpa wants you to
                be strong, and he is watching over you.

VAL   *[Sign]* Is it okay with you if I bring the picture
                with me?

HUMPHREY   *[Sign]* Of course you can. It is time for your
                bath before we get ready to go out.

VAL   *[Sign]* Okay, thanks for finding the picture. I
                need it.

HUMPHREY   *[Sign]* No problem, you are welcome.

The Humphrey family and Val go to the steakhouse. While they eat dinner, Val is quiet and looks at the picture of his grandpa as the Humphrey's watch him.

VAL   *(Eats meatloaf)* *[Sign]* Humphrey, I am done with
                supper. It was very good, thanks so much for
                bringing me here.

HUMPHREY   *[Sign]* You are welcome, I am glad you liked it.
                What kind of dessert do you want?

VAL   *[Sign]* I want a milkshake.

HUMPHREY   *[Sign]* I am sorry, they don't have milkshakes.

VAL	*[Sign]* Can we go to McDonald's to get one?
CW	*[Voice]* Sure, let's go to McDonald's to get a milkshake.
HUMPHREY	*[Voice]* CW, how sweet of you.
CW	*[Voice]* I think his grandpa would want this.
HUMPHREY	*(Smiles) [Voice]* Thanks, CW.
CW	*[Voice]* Ask Val what kind of milkshake he likes.
HUMPHREY	*(Turns to Val) [Sign]* Which one do you want?
VAL	*[Sign]* Brown.
HUMPHREY	*[Sign and voice]* Brown? Wait, he wants chocolate.
VAL	*[Sign]* I think of Grandpa when I drink milkshakes.
HUMPHREY	*[Sign]* I know you do. He is happy seeing you drink a milkshake.
VAL	*[Sign]* I miss Grandpa.

After McDonalds, Val and the Humphrey family go to the mall. Thomas wants to go to the toy store, but Val wants to go to the flower shop instead.

THOMAS	*[Voice]* Let's go to the toy store!
VAL	*[Sign]* I want flowers.
HUMPHREY	*[Sign]* Why do you want flowers?
VAL	*[Sign]* I want to give them to my grandma. She is sad and will miss Grandpa.
HUMPHREY	*[Sign]* That's a good idea, let's send them to

her, from you.

VAL	*[Sign]* I want to add your name, too.
HUMPHREY	*[Sign]* Why?
VAL	*[Sign]* Remember, she baked an apple pie for all of you.
HUMPHREY	*[Sign to Val and voice to her family]* Oh, I remember. Is it okay with CW and the boys?
CW	*[Voice]* Of course, the apple pie was very delicious.
HUMPHREY	*[Voice and sign]* Okay, the flowers are from Val and the Humphreys.

The flower man arrives at the Woodburn residence and delivers flowers to Val's grandma.

DELIEVERY MAN	*[Voice]* Hello, is Merle Woodburn here? I am here to deliver flowers to her.
BETTY	*[Voice]* Thanks so much. I will give them to her.
GRANDMA	*[Voice]* Pretty roses, I wonder who sent them to me.
BETTY	*[Voice]* Here is a card.
GRANDMA	*(Reads the card)* *[Voice]* Aww, it is from the Humphreys and Val, I am glad he stayed with them. I need to talk to them and say thanks.
BETTY	*[Voice]* Okay, I am going to call Mary Sue now.

The phone rings and Humphrey picks it up.

HUMPHREY	*[Voice]* Hello, this is the Humphrey residence.

BETTY	*[Voice]* Hello Mary Sue, it is me. I am very sorry that I haven't called you for a while. The funeral was beautiful, but very sad.
HUMPHREY	*[Voice]* Hello Betty, it is okay. I know it must be rough on you. Did your mother get the flowers from us?
BETTY	*[Voice]* Yes, she loves them. She was very sad that Val was not here, but I told her you would take care of him. What is Val doing today?
HUMPHREY	*[Voice]* He is playing board games with the boys; he is doing fine now.
BETTY	*[Voice]* Good, how was he after you told him about his grandpa?
HUMPHREY	*[Voice]* He was very sad, but we comforted him. I found a picture of Grandpa and him in his suitcase. He took it when we went to eat out.
BETTY	*[Voice]* Great, you did a good job with him. When is Val going back to school?
HUMPHREY	*[Voice]* The students won't arrive until Monday, I will take him with me. Will all of you be home next weekend?
BETTY	*[Voice]* Yes, we will be.
HUMPHREY	*[Voice]* Great, we are thinking of you and your family and we keep praying. I better let you go spend time with your mother.
BETTY	*[Voice]* Wait, Mama wants to speak to you. She wants to say thank you so much for taking care of her grandson.

HUMPHREY   *[Voice]* Okay, I would love to hear from her.

GRANDMA   *[Voice]* This is Val's grandmother. Thanks so
                  much for sending flowers to me. It made me
                  think about Val. I am sad that he is not here,
                  but I am glad you are taking care of him for us.

HUMPHREY   *[Voice]* Oh Mrs. Woodburn, you are welcome.
                  Val keeps asking about you, it was his idea to
                  send the flowers to you. He is doing a little
                  better. You are in our thoughts and prayers.

GRANDMA   *[Voice]* Thanks so much, I appreciate it. Can
                  you put Val on the phone please?

HUMPHREY   *[Voice]* Excuse me? But he can't hear your
                  voice.

GRAMDMA   *[Voice]* Let him hold the phone, so he can feel
                  my voice.

HUMPHREY   *[Voice]* Let me get Val. Just a minute. Boys!
                  Send Val here. His grandma wants to talk to
                  him.

The boys show up and Val looks at Humphrey.

VAL   *[Sign]* Who is on the phone?

HUMPHREY   *[Sign]* Grandma, she wants to talk to you.

THOMAS   *[Voice]* But he can't hear her voice.

HUMPHREY   *[Voice]* I know, but he can feel her voice on the
                  phone. Please hold the phone so you can feel
                  your grandma's voice.

GRANDMA   *[Voice]* Val, I love and miss you so much!

VAL   *(In tears)* *[Sign]* I can feel her voice.

HUMPHREY   *[Sign]* Great! She said she loves and misses you so much.

Scene Nineteen: Val and Humphrey Say Goodbye

The next morning Humphrey takes Val back to Vestal Hall, but he is not sure if he is ready for school or not. Humphrey comforts him.

VAL   *[Sign]* Do I have to go back to school?

HUMPHREY   *[Sign]* Yes, the weather is back to normal.

VAL   *[Sign]* I am too sad to be here.

HUMPHREY   *[Sign]* I know you miss Grandpa, but he wants you to go back to school and be strong.

VAL   *[Sign]* He is watching over me?

HUMPHREY   *[Sign]* That's right. Your houseparent is waiting for you. I need to go back to class for a meeting.

VAL   *[Sign]* Wait, I wanted to say thank you so much for taking me to your place. I had a good time with all of you. I appreciate your support.

HUMPHREY   *[Sign]* Oh, you are always welcome. You know how much we love you. We will see each other again.

VAL   *[Sign]* I love you too. Wait.

HUMPHREY   *[Sign]* What?

VAL   *(Hugs her) [Sign]* I almost forgot to hug you. I will never forget you.

HUMPHREY   *[Sign]* Neither will I.

Val smiles and walks to Vestal Hall.

HUMPHREY   *(In tears) [Voice]* I will never forget you. You
                  will always be my favorite student!

*Val looks around and watches as Humphrey walks to Eagles Hall. He has
flashbacks of their time together. He is in tears as he goes into Vestal Hall.*

Fade Out

Val Melvin continued his education at ENCSD until 1988. He graduated with a high school diploma and became a member of the National Honor Society. He graduated from Wake Technical Community College, with a Computer Business Associate's Degree. He had several operations over the years. His mandible was normal after the conclusion of surgical procedures that began immediately following his birth and continued until 1999.

Mary Sue Humphrey continued to teach at Eagles Hall until she retired in 1996. She was widowed and is the grandmother of six grandchildren. She was reunited with her favorite student, Val, at his 40th birthday party.

THE END

To Traci

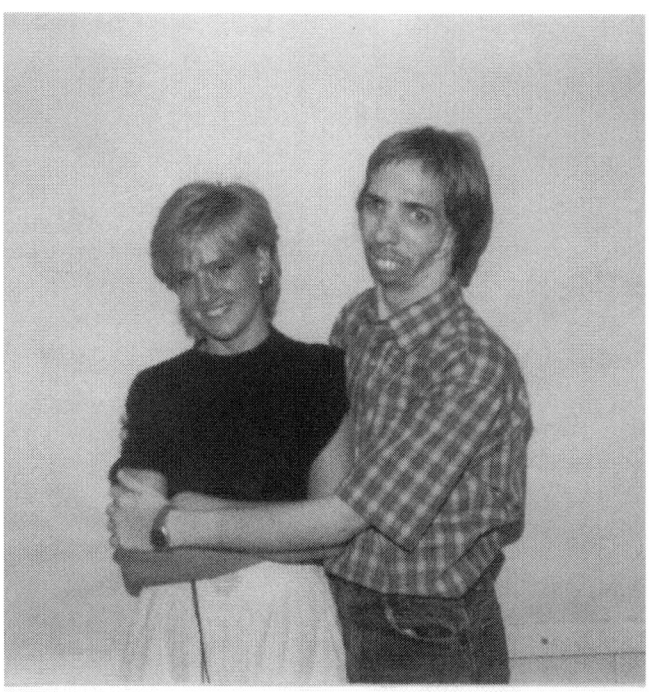

This book is in the loving memory of my classmate and my dear close friend, Traci Lynn Baines. We were in the same class at Eagles Hall. We were separated at Vestal Hall, but we still saw each other. We were very close in high school, and we graduated together in 1988. She was like the sister I never had. I still miss her and love her as I always did.

Epilogue

I had many wonderful moments with Mrs. Humphrey when I was in her class. I hoped she would be my teacher again in the next school year, but I found out my new teacher would be Clara Eatmon, who taught first grade. I had a hard time accepting her until Humphrey told me that she and I shared the same birthday: July 30th. I also realized I had the same classmates that I had in Humphrey's class and I was able to accept the change. I missed Mrs. Humphrey when I was in Eatmon's class, but I knew I had to listen to what Eatmon said, so Humphrey would be proud of me. Clara Eatmon was very different from Mary Sue Humphrey, but she learned how to teach me. She treated me well, like Humphrey did. I learned everything from her; we went on some field trips like to the airport, the pumpkin patch, and to Raleigh.

I remember when Mrs. Eatmon went to the classroom to decorate for winter on a Sunday and she invited me to help her. She was very wise. When my mother brought cupcakes for my class, Mrs. Eatmon said I could bring some to Mrs. Humphrey's class. I enjoyed making her class very happy. Eatmon invited me and my classmates to her house for a cookout and I met her husband and her sons, who were very nice. I gave Eatmon some flowers on the last day of school.

When I came back to ENCSD from the summer of 1978, I had moved to Vestal Hall for the second grade. I was uncomfortable there because of the older kids, and I missed Mrs. Cole and Mrs. Humphrey. Mrs. Sutton was originally my second grade teacher with the same classmates, but the Vestal Hall principal moved me to another classroom. The teacher was Sue Dail and the classmates were much older than I was. My parents were not happy with this change. I liked Sue Dail and she reminded me of Mrs. Humphrey because she was very protective of me. She taught me many things and she comforted me during my grandfather's death. I enjoyed her teaching. She took me to her place for dinner with her family. Like Humphrey, Sue Dail was very worried about my chewing and would watch me eat.

She was my teacher again for the third grade, but my classmates were very different, though they were nice to me. The incident with the sausage, which I mentioned before, actually happened when I was in Sue Dail's class. I had a rough time swallowing the sausage, and Sue Dail called for help. Gary Farmer and James Massey helped me go to the infirmary and the nurses got the sausage out of my mouth. Sue Dail kept checking on me and fixed oatmeal for me. I know Sue Dail was a very caring and loving teacher, she did an amazing job teaching me. While in her class, I stopped wearing a trach, so the suction machine was sent home. I still went to the infirmary to brush my teeth and I had a small hole in my neck, but with the suction machine gone, I began to ride the bus with the other students in January 1979.

I wanted Dail to be my teacher again, but the fourth grade teacher was Mamie Boyette. She was very different from my previous teachers. She taught us math and government, and we even took a trip on a train. Boyette did a great job teaching and taught me something very interesting: the solar system. We learned about the nine planets and their moons, and how they orbit around the sun. In 2006, Pluto was removed from the solar system and was demoted as the dwarf planet because it was very different from the other planets. Boyette gave me an award for math that year.

My sixth grade teacher was Jackie Simmons. She was very sweet and beautiful, I had a crush on her. She was not pleased with my grades because I daydreamed in class. I drew a lot, but it hurt my grades. I thought she didn't like me at all, but when I admitted to her that I liked her so much, she told me to keep working hard for her and said no daydreaming. After that, my grades improved and she was very proud of me. She hugged me after class and invited me me to eat pizza with her because I had listened to what she said. She had a tragedy when her oldest son died. She grieved for him for several months. I couldn't stop thinking about her and wanted to cheer her up. I did her Christmas drama twice to make her happy. Later, she had two more children.

My seventh grade teacher was Nannie Murray. She was very nice, but she didn't like the word lie; she was a good Christian. She complained when someone signed lie; she wanted us to sign false instead. When Murray found out my father was a pastor, she began to be extra nice to me and taught me about being honest.

Murray was my homeroom teacher in my senior year, but she passed away before graduation. She was not my only teacher in the seventh grade; John Farmer taught us reading, and Ricky Masten taught us science. Mr. Masten and I grew closer when he taught me. I spent time with him and his family in the summer. We would talk about the solar system a lot. My gym teacher, Gary Farmer, was very nice to me after a talk with my father. I was not good at sports, but he asked me to be his scorekeeper when the students played games like baseball, hockey, and volleyball.

During my last year of Vestal Hall, I missed my first three weeks of school because my jaws were wired. Gena Andrews tutored me until I got back to school. Jean Watson was my homeroom teacher for the eighth grade and she taught us my favorite subject: math. Patricia Nooe (formerly Miss Ezzard) taught reading, Lawrence Seeger taught North Carolina history, and Audrey Morgan taught language. We had some classes at the vocational building for the last period. Ricky Masten taught science. I was very happy to have him as my teacher, and I was very pleased to have Jean Watson as my math teacher. She was very sweet and kind to me. We had wonderful moments in the eighth grade. That school year was the final year for my Vestal Hall principal, Elva Evans, and we had a retirement party for her.

We were looking forward to high school at McAdams Hall, but everything changed when the students from CNCSD moved to ENCSD because their school didn't have a high school program. Freshman year, my two favorite teachers were Joel Brame, the math teacher, and Freida Humphrey, the English teacher, because they were very sweet and funny. Sophomore year was okay for me, Barbara Curtis taught my computer class and I learned how to type from Mrs. Godwin. Junior year was good, I took driver's education with Don Webb, and learned how to cook with Mrs. Stone.

Senior year was my best year because the students were nicer to me than they were in the previous years. I didn't have to take a math class, and my reading class was very easy. I missed school for two months due to my back operation, and Debra Davis tutored me at home. I became a member of the National Honor Society and graduated with a High School diploma. Some of my old teachers were there and congratulated me. ENCSD was like a second home to me.

I had many operations at Duke Hospital during my childhood years. My parents worked hard with the doctors to improve my health and appearance. My parents asked my doctor about operations during the summer break because they didn't want me to skip any school days. I had many appointments with my doctor during my school years. Several people in my life, including Mary Sue Humphrey and her husband, visited me at the hospital. My parents explained to me why I needed the operations, but I got very tired of it.

The last year I had an operation at Duke Hospital was in 1986, because some of my doctors retired. I was sad to leave Duke Hospital, but I remained a Duke fan. During my senior year of high school I had back surgery at Durham Regional Hospital. I was forced to stay home for two months for my recovery. I returned to ENCSD on January 1988 and I was not allowed to lift heavy things. After my graduation, I had a serious operation in Boston, where I stayed for one month. I enjoyed viewing Boston, but my operation wasn't successful.

I was transferred to Carolina Medical Center in Charlotte. My doctor was Dr. Matthew, and he did an amazing job fixing my jaws. In 1999, I finally had my neck sutured so I could swim in the lake. Dr. Matthew told my parents to send me to Wisconsin, where I met Dr. Julie Brown. She made a left ear which looks real. I am very blessed that I don't have any more operations. I am thankful for all the doctors and nurses who cared for me during my many operations.

After I graduated from high school, I went to Craven County Community College to study computer business programing. I moved to Raleigh after living in New Bern for 17 years. I continued my education at Wake Tech; I had to try several times to graduate because operations interrupted my class years. In August 1995, I finally graduated from Wake Tech Community College with an associate's degree. My brother got married one month later, and he and his wife, Allison, have two beautiful children, Joseph and Emily. I am a proud uncle. I worked at the Department of Revenue in Raleigh for 14 years. I enjoy swimming and riding my bicycle. I keep in touch with my friends from ENCSD. My life is getting better, I am so proud of my accomplishments. I have had many physical barriers to overcome to become the man that I am.

ENCSD

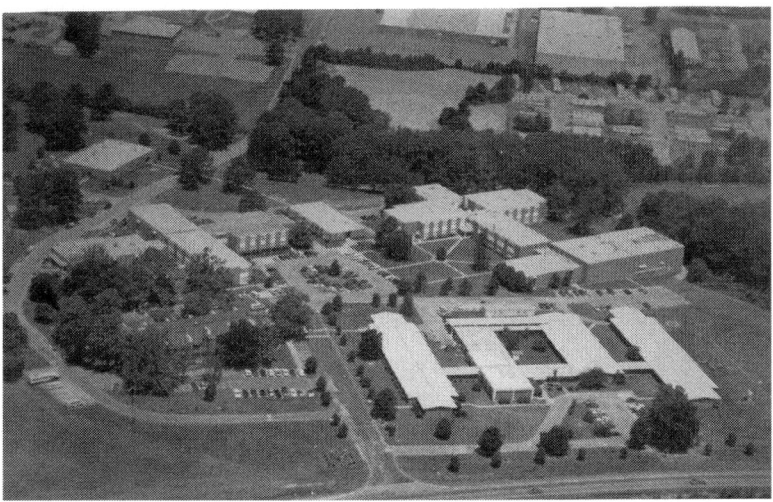

Eastern North Carolina School for the Deaf was established in 1964. The first superintendent was Ronald McAdams, who served until 1980. The high school program began in 1979, and the high school building was named after him. The school's mascot is The Hornet, and its colors are green and gold.

Eagles Hall is the building in front; it is where Mrs. Humphrey taught me. It is the first building I lived in at school and I stayed there for three years.

Woodard Hall is to the left of Eagles Hall; the infirmary was on the second floor and the faculty offices were on the first floor. As a kid, I walked to the infirmary from Eagles Hall to Woodard Hall.

Vestal Hall is in the back, on the left; it is where I lived after Eagles Hall. I stayed there for six years, during middle school.

McAdams Hall is in the back and to the right; it is where I stayed during my four years of high school.

Mayfield Hall, between Vestal Hall and McAdams Hall, was used as a vocational building until Alford Vocational Building (upper left) was built in 1983. When I was in high school, Mayfield Hall housed classrooms for students with special needs.

A lot has changed since I graduated. A new building was added, Eagles Hall has been closed, and its playground is also gone.

Teachers During My ENCSD Years

Eagles Hall

Principal: Sandra Simmons

Ann Barnes	K-Prep II	1975-1976
Mary Sue Humphrey	K-Prep III	1976-1977
Clara Eatmon	First Grade	1977-1978

Vestal Hall

Principal: Elva Evans

Sue Dail	Second Grade	1978-1979
Sue Dail	Third Grade	1979-1980
Mamie Boyette	Fourth Grade	1980-1981
Jackie Simmons	Sixth Grade	1981-1982
Nannie Murray	Seventh Grade	1982-1983
Jean Watson	Eighth Grade	1983-1984

McAdams Hall

Principal: Brenda Farmer

Marion Parris*	Freshman	1984-1985
Jasmine Albertson*	Sophomore	1985-1986
Jackie Mullins*	Junior	1986-1987
Nannie Murray*	Senior	1987-1988

*These were my homeroom teachers throughout high school.

Made in the USA
Columbia, SC
22 March 2021

34278319R00154